NEUROLOGY CLINICAL PRACTICE AND CRITICAL CARE

By. Stuhan Davis

ISBN: 9781688255326

2012 Edition

Disclaimer
Iin view of the rapid changes occurring in medical science, as well as the possibility of human error, this site may contain technical inaccuracies, typographical or other errors. It is the responsibility of the reading physician who must rely on experience and knowledge about the patient to determine the best treatment and care pathway. The information contained herein is provided "as is", without warranty of any kind. The contributors to this book, disclaim responsibility for any errors or omissions or for results obtained from the use of information contained herein.

Prologue

Neurointensive care is a relatively new field that has developed as a subspecialty of critical care and neurology. The goal of neurointensive care, and the neurointensivist, is to treat and prevent primary and secondary brain (or other nervous system) injury. Inherent in this goal are the monitoring tools unique to the neurointensive care unit, including the most basic but perhaps the most important tool, the neurologic examination. In the era of the subspecialty of critical care neurology, the neurologist is working now as an aggressive interventionalist who manages life-threatening disorders of the nervous system. The neurointensivist's role is to help follow the neurologic status and treat the patient while integrating his/her knowledge of other organ systems and expertise in critical care, to provide the most comprehensive care possible for the patient.

Critical care neurology is practiced in emergency rooms, in consultations in general medical and surgical intensive care units, in intermediary care units such as stroke units, and in specialized neurointensive care units where patients are frequently on life-support systems involving ventilators, intravascular lines, and monitoring and treatment devices. Data has shown that care provided by clinicians specializing in neurologic injury, and within dedicated neurointensive care units, improves patient functional outcome, and reduces hospital mortality, length of stay and resource utilization.

This book emphasizes the clinical and practical aspects of management in the neurointensive care unit.

This book is written, mainly, for the neurologist working in, or directing, a specialized neurointensive care unit (neurointensivists), as well as other specialists including stroke neurologists, neurosurgeons, pulmonary/critical care specialists, anesthesiologists, nurse practitioners, critical care registered

nurses, and therapists all working together towards improved neurologic recovery.

We hope this book can provide a new addition to the emerging literature of critical care neurology, and heighten the recognition by general medical and surgical intensivists of the importance and complexities of nervous system dysfunction in critically ill and injured patients.

Editors

Nabil Kitchener, MD, PhD Professor of Neurology, GOTHI, Egypt
President of Egyptian Cerebro- Cardio-Vascular Association (ECCVA) and Board Director of World Stroke Organization (WSO)
www.ECCVA.com nabilkitchener@consultant.com

Saher Hashem, MD Professor and Chairman of Neurology and Neurocritical Department
Cairo University, Egypt

Mervat Wahba, MD, FCCP Assistant Professor of Neurology Department of Neurology University of Tennessee Health Sciences Center, UTHSC, USA

Authors

Magdy Khalaf, MD
Consultant Neurologist and Chairman of Neurocritical Care Unit
GOTHI, Egypt

Bassem Zarif, MD
Lecturer of Cardiology
National Heart Institute, GOTHI, Egypt

Simin Mansoor, MD Department of Neurology University of Tennessee Health Sciences Center, UTHSC, USA

Table of Contents

TABLE OF CONTENTS	**1**
1. ASSESSMENT OF PATIENTS IN NEUROLOGICAL EMERGENCY	**5**
Physical Exam	**8**
1. Mental status	8
2. Cranial nerve (CN) exam	8
3. Motor exam	10
4. Reflexes	10
5. Sensory exam	10
6. Coordination and balance	10
7. Neuroanatomical localization	11
Brain	11
Spinal cord	11
Conclusions	**12**
2. HOW TO APPROACH AN UNCONSCIOUS PATIENT	**13**
Basic assessments	16
General Care of the Comatose Patient	**19**
Permanent Vegetative State	**20**
Diagnosis	21
Management	21
Locked-in Syndrome	**23**
Brain Death	**24**

3. DOCUMENTATION AND SCORES 25

Delirium 31

4. BRAIN INJURIES 33

Types of Brain Injuries 33
    Primary brain injuries 33
    Secondary brain injuries 36

Management of Special Issues 38
    Traumatic brain injury 38
    Acute stroke 40
    Status epilepticus (SE) 41
    Neuromuscular emergencies 42
    Management of subarachnoid hemorrhage 45

5. BASIC HEMODYNAMIC MONITORING OF NEUROCRITICAL PATIENTS 48

6. NEUROCRITICAL MONITORING 54

Clinical Assessment 55
    The Glasgow Coma Scale 55
    Pupillary response 55

Invasive Monitoring 56
    Measuring ICP 57
    Indications for ICP monitoring 57
    Intracranial Pressure Waveforms and Analysis 58
    Jugular Venous Oximetry ($SjvO_2$) 62
    Insertion of Jugular Venous Saturation Catheter: Insertion 63
    Indications for $SjvO_2$ Monitoring: 63
    Interpretation of Changes in $SjvO_2$: 64
    Brain Tissue Oximetry 65
    Direct measures of CBF: 65
    Xenon-Enhanced CT: 65
    SPECT (Single Photo Emission CT): 66

Noninvasive Monitoring	66
Continuous measures of CBF by Transcranial Doppler	66
Technique for Insonating the Middle Cerebral Artery	67
Near Infrared Spectroscopy	68
Electrophysiological Monitoring	69
Continuous Electroencephalogram Monitoring: When a	70
Application of the EEG in the ICU:	71
Multimodal Monitoring	72
Conclusions	74

7. CEREBRAL EDEMA 75

Management of Cerebral Edema 79

8. GENERAL NEUROLOGICAL TREATMENT 80

STRATEGIES 80

Swallowing Disturbances 81

Respiratory Management in Neurocritical Care 82

Infection Control in Neurocritical Care 85

Pain Relief and Sedation	87
Bedside approach to the agitated patient	88

Role of Rehabilitation 89

Diagnostic Findings in Cerebral Death 90

Conclusion 93

9. MEDICAL DISEASES AND METABOLIC

ENCEPHALOPATHIES 94

Examination of the Encephalopathic Patient 95

General Pathophysiology 96

Hepatic Encephalopathy 96
Complications of hepatic encephalopathy (HE) 97
Treatment of hepatic encephalopathy 99

Renal Encephalopathies 99

Fluid and Electrolyte Imbalance 101
Osmolarity disorders 101
Syndrome of inappropriate secretion of antidiuretic 102

Encephalopathy in Diabetic Patients 103
Nonketotic hyperosmolar hyperglycemia (NHH): Usually 103

Hypoxic Ischemic Encephalopathy (HIE) 104

Septic Encephalopathy 105

Drug-induced Encephalopathies 105

10. REFERENCES 106

1. Assessment of Patients in Neurological Emergency
NAbil Kitchener, SAher HAshem

Care in specialized intensive care units (ICUs) is generally of higher quality than in general care units. Neurocritical care focuses on the care of critically ill patients with primary or secondary neurosurgical and neurological problems and was initially developed to manage postoperative neurosurgical patients. It expanded thereafter to the management of patients with traumatic brain injury (TBI), intracranial hemorrhage and complications of subarachnoid hemorrhage; including vasospasm, elevated intracranial pressure (ICP) and the cardiopulmonary complications of brain injury.

Neurocritical care units have developed to coordinate the management of critically ill neurological patients in a single specialized unit, which includes many clinical domains. Care is provided by a multidisciplinary team trained to recognize and deal with the unique aspects of the neurological disease processes, as several treatable neurological disorders are characterized by imminent risk of severe and irreversible neurological injury or death if treatment is delayed.

Some diseases need immediate action, so admission to the NICU is the best solution when there is:

1) Impaired level of consciousness.
2) Progressive respiratory impairment or the need for mechanical ventilation in a neurological patient.
3) Status epilepticus or prolonged seizures.
4) Clinical or Computed Tomographic (CT) evidence of

raised Intracranial Pressure (ICP), whatever the cause (space occupying lesion, cerebral edema or hemorrhagic conversion of a cerebral infarct, intracerebral hemorrhage, etc.)
5) Need for monitoring (for example, level of consciousness, ICP, continuous electroencephalography (cEEG)), and
6) Need for specific treatments (Baldwin 2010) (e.g., neurosurgery, intravenous or arterial thrombolysis).

In the Neurocritical Care unit, patients with primary neurological diseases such as myasthenia gravis, Guillain-Barré syndrome, status epilepticus, and stroke have a better outcome than those patients with secondary neurological diseases. So, we can conclude that these specialized units have greater experience in the anticipation, early recognition, and management of potentially fatal complications.

Early identification of patients at risk of life threatening neurological illness in order to manage them properly and to prevent further deterioration is the role of general assessment of new patients in a neurological emergency. History taking and a rapid neurological assessment of a specific patient in specialized neurocritical care units helps answer the question 'how sick is this patient?'.

The neurologic screening examination in the emergency settings focuses primarily on identifying acute, potentially life- threatening processes, and secondarily on identifying disorders that require other opinions, of other specialists.

The importance of urgent neurologic assessment comes from recent advances in the management of neurologic disorders needing timely intervention like thrombolysis in acute ischemic

stroke, anticonvulsants for nonconvulsive and subtle generalized status epilepticus, and plasmapheresis for

Guillain-Barré, etc.

It is obvious that interventions can be time-sensitive and can significantly reduce morbidity and mortality.

A comprehensive neurologic screening assessment can be accomplished within minutes if performed in an organized and systematic manner (Goldberg 1987). Neurologic screening assessment includes six major components of the neurologic exam, namely:
1) Mental status
2) Cranial nerve exam
3) Motor exam
4) Reflexes
5) Sensory exam
6) Evaluation of coordination and balance.

Based on the chief findings of the screening assessment, further evaluation or investigations can be then decided upon.

History

A careful history is the first step to successful diagnosis, and then intervention. Careful history provides clues to the pathology of the patient's condition, and may help direct the diagnostic workup. For example, an alert patient with a headache associated with neck pain that started after a car accident might help direct the examination and radiographic imaging to focus on cervical spine injury or neck vessels (carotid or vertebral artery) dissection, while the same patient not in a car accident may direct your attention to a spontaneous subarachnoid hemorrhage.

The history begins with a definition of the patient's complaint, but aiming at determining key points: time and mode of onset, mode of progression, associated symptoms, and a prior history of similar conditions. Dramatic or acute onset of neurologic events suggests a vascular insult and mandates immediate attention and intervention.

Physical Exam

1. Mental status

Usually we start neurologic examination by assessing the patient's mental status (Strub 2000).

A full mental status exam is not necessary in the patient who is conscious, awake, oriented, and conversant; on the contrary it must be fully investigated in patients with altered mental status.

Sometimes, we can find no change in mental status; at that point careful consideration should be given to concerns of family.

A systematic approach to the assessment of mental status is helpful in detecting acute as well as any chronic disease, such as delirious state in a demented patient (Lewis 1995). The CAM (confusion assessment method) score was developed to assist in diagnosing delirium in different contexts. CAM assesses four components: acute onset, inattention, disorganized thinking or an altered level of consciousness with a fluctuating course. A 'Mini-Mental Status' test can also be used but usually is reserved for patients with suspected cognitive dysfunction as it evaluates five domains – orientation, registration, attention, recall, and language (Strub 2000).

2. Cranial nerve (CN) exam

Cranial Nerves II - VIII function testing are of utmost value in the neurologic assessment in an emergency setting (Monkhouse 2006).

Cranial Nerves II – Optic nerve assessment involves visual acuity and fields, along with a fundus exam and a swinging flashlight test. Visual field exam using the confrontation method is rapid and reliable. Visual loss in one eye suggests a nerve lesion, i.e., in front of the chiasm; bitemporal hemianopsia suggests a lesion at the optic chiasm; a quadrant deficit suggests a lesion in the optic tracts; bilateral visual loss suggests cortical disease.

Assessment of the optic disc, retinal arteries, and retinal veins can be done by a fundus exam, to discover papilledema, flame hemorrhages or sheathing.

Cranial Nerves III, IV, VI – CN III innervates the extraocular muscles for primarily adduction and vertical gaze. CN III function is tested in conjunction with IV, which aids in internal depression via the superior oblique, and VI, which controls abduction via the lateral rectus. Extraocular muscle function is tested for diplopia, which requires binocular vision and thus will resolve when one eye is occluded. Marked nystagmus on lateral gaze or any nystagmus on vertical gaze is abnormal; vertical nystagmus is seen in brainstem lesions or intoxication, while pendular nystagmus is generally a congenital condition.

The pupillary light reflex is mediated via the parasympathetic nerve fibers running on the outside of CN III. In the swinging flashlight test a light is shone from one eye to the other; when the light is shone directly into a normal eye, both eyes constrict via the direct and the consensual light response.

Pupillary size must be documented. Asymmetry in pupils of less than 1 mm is not significant. Significant difference in pupil size suggests nerve compression due to aneurysms or due to cerebral herniation, in patients with altered mental status.

Bilateral pupillary dilation is seen with prolonged anoxia or due to drugs (anticholinergics), while bilateral pupillary constriction is seen with pontine hemorrhage or as the result of drugs (e.g., opiates, clonidine).

Cranial Nerve V – Individual branch testing of the trigeminal nerve is unnecessary, as central nervous system lesions affecting CN V usually involve all three branches.

Cranial Nerve VII – The facial nerve innervates motor function to the face, and sensory function to the ear canal, as well as to the anterior two-thirds of the tongue. Central lesions cause contralateral weakness of the face muscles below the eyes. **Cranial Nerve VIII** – The acoustic nerve has a vestibular and a cochlear component. An easy screening test for hearing defects is accomplished by speaking in graded volumes to the patient.

When vestibular nerve defects are suspected, patients are assessed for nystagmus, via a past-pointing test and a positive response to the Nylen-Barany maneuver.

3. Motor exam

Motor system assessment focuses on detecting asymmetric strength deficits, which may indicate an acute CNS lesion. Testing motor power can be difficult or impossible in the uncooperative patient. It is not mandatory to test different muscle groups but instead just test for the presence of a "drift". In diseased patients, the hand and arm on the affected side will slowly drift or pronate when they try to hold their arm out horizontally, palms up with eyes closed.

4. Reflexes

For rapid assessment of reflexes, major deep tendon reflexes and the plantar reflex must be elicited. Major deep tendon reflexes include the patellar reflex, the Achilles reflex, the biceps reflex, and the triceps reflex. Response can be graded from 0 (no reflex) to 4+ (hyperreflexia). Asymmetrical reflexes are the most important as they are considered pathologic. Many reflexes indicate upper motor neuron disease; the most commonly elicited is Babinski's reflex.

5. Sensory exam

For rapid assessment of the sensory system, pain and light touch sensations should be done. Testing for other sensory modalities is reserved for patients with suspected neuropathies or for further evaluation of sensory complaints.

6. Coordination and balance

Coordination depends on functional integration of the cerebellum and sensory input from vision, proprioception, and the vestibular sense. Coordination assessment is an important part of neurological assessment, as many central lesions may present only with coordination disturbance, such as cerebellar infarction, hemorrhage or cerebellar connections insult.

By the end of the examination, you should reach a clinical diagnosis, which includes answers to the two critical questions, what is the lesion? and where is the lesion?

7. Neuroanatomical localization

Some knowledge of neuroanatomy is essential for correct localization. The first step in localizing neurological lesions should be to determine if it is a central (upper motor neuron) lesion (i.e., in the brain or spinal cord) versus a peripheral (lower motor neuron) lesion (i.e., nerve or muscle).

The hallmark of **upper motor neuron lesions** is hyperreflexia with or without increased muscle tone. Central (upper motor neuron) lesions are localized to:

Brain
– Cortical brain (frontal, temporal, parietal, or occipital lobes)
– Subcortical brain structures (corona radiata, internal capsule, basal ganglia, or thalamus)
– Brainstem (medulla, pons, or midbrain)
– Cerebellum

Spinal cord
– Cervicomedullary junction
– Cervical
– Thoracic
– Upper lumbar

The hallmark of a **lower motor neuron (LMN) lesion** is decreased muscle tone, leading to flaccidity and hyporeflexia. Peripheral LMN lesions are localized to:

- Anterior horn cells
- Nerve root(s)
- Plexus
- Peripheral nerve
- Neuromuscular junction
- Muscle

Conclusions

1. The neurological screening examination provides the clinician with the necessary data to make management decisions.
2. A cranial nerve examination gives plenty of data in the emergency setting and is a critical component of the screening exam.

2. How to Approach an Unconscious Patient

MAGdy KhALAf, NABil Kitchener

Coma (from the Greek κώμα [koma], meaning deep sleep) is a state of unconsciousness lasting more than 6 hours, in which a person cannot be awakened, fails to respond normally to painful stimuli, light or sound, lacks a normal sleep-wake cycle and does not initiate voluntary actions.

All unconscious patients should have neurological examinations to help determine the site and nature of the lesion, to monitor progress, and to determine prognosis. Neurological examination is most useful in the well-oxygenated, normotensive, normoglycemic patient with no sedation, since hypoxia, hypotension, hypoglycemia and sedating drugs profoundly affect the signs elicited. Therefore, immediate therapeutic intervention is a must to correct aberrations of hypoxia, hypercarbia and hypoglycemia. Medications recently taken that cause unconsciousness or delirium must be identified quickly followed by rapid clinical assessment to detect the form of coma either with or without lateralizing signs, with or without signs of meningeal irritation, the pattern of breathing, the size and reactivity of pupils and ocular movements, the motor response, the airway clearance, the pattern of breathing and circulation integrity, etc.

Special consideration must be given to neurological causes which may lead to unconsciousness like status epilepticus (either convulsive or non-convulsive), locked-in state, persistent vegetative state and lastly brain stem death. Any disturbances of thermoregulation must be measured.

Coma may result from a variety of conditions including intoxication, metabolic abnormalities, central nervous system diseases, acute neurologic injuries such as stroke, hypoxia or traumatic injuries including head trauma caused by falls or vehicle collisions. Looking for the pathogenesis of coma, two important neurological components must function perfectly that maintain consciousness. The first is the gray matter covering the outer layer of the brain and the other is a structure located in the brainstem called the reticular activating system (RAS or ARAS), a more primitive structure that is in close connection with the reticular formation (RF), a critical anatomical structure needed for maintenance of arousal. It is necessary to investigate the integrity of the bilateral cerebral cortices and the reticular activating system (RAS), as a rule. Unilateral hemispheric lesions do not produce stupor and coma unless they are of a mass sufficient to compress either the contralateral hemisphere or the brain stem (Bateman 2001). Metabolic disorders impair consciousness by diffuse effects on both the reticular formation and the cerebral cortex. Coma is rarely a permanent state although less than 10% of patients survive coma without significant disability (Bateman 2001); for ICU patients with persistent coma, the outcome is grim.

Maneuvers to be established with an unconscious patient include cardiopulmonary resuscitation, laboratory investigations, a radiological examination to recognize brain edema, as well as any skull, cervical, spinal, chest, and multiple traumas. Intracranial pressure and neurophysiological monitoring are important new areas for investigation in the unconscious patient.

Diagnosis

In the initial assessment of coma, it is common to judge by

spontaneous actions, response to vocal stimuli and response to painful stimuli; this is known as the AVPU (alert, vocal stimuli, painful stimuli, unconscious) scale. The most common scales used for rapid assessment are:

1. The Glasgow Coma Scale (GCS), which aims to record the conscious state of a person, in initial as well as continuing assessment. When a patient is assessed and the resulting score is either 14 (original scale) or 15 (the more widely used modified or revised scale), this means 'normal'; while if a patient is unable to voluntarily open their eyes, does not have a sleep-wake cycle, is unresponsive in spite of strong sensory (painful) or verbal stimuli and who generally scores between 3 to 8 on the Glasgow Coma Scale, (s)he is considered to be in coma.

2. Pediatric Glasgow Coma Scale: The Pediatric Glasgow Coma Scale (PGCS) is the equivalent of the Glasgow Coma Scale used to assess the mental state of adult patients. As with the GCS, the PGCS comprises three tests: eye, verbal and motor responses. The three values separately as well as their sum are considered (Holmes 2005). The lowest possible PGCS is 3 (deep coma or death) whilst the highest is 15 (fully awake and aware) (Holmes 2005).

Diagnosis of coma is simple; but determining the cause of the underlying pathology may prove to be challenging. As in those with deep unconsciousness, there is a risk of asphyxiation as control over the muscles in the face and throat is diminished, so those in a coma are typically assessed for airway management, nasopharyngeal airway or endotracheal intubation to safeguard the airway (Formisano 2004).

Following the previous assessment patients with impaired consciousness can be classified according to their degree of consciousness disturbance into lethargic, stuporous or comatose. **Lethargy** resembles sleepiness, except that the patient is incapable of becoming fully alert; these patients are conversant and attentive but slow to respond, unable to adequately perform simple concentration tasks such as counting from 20 to 1, or reciting the months in reverse.

Stupor means incomplete arousal to painful stimuli, little or no response to verbal commands, the patient may obey commands temporarily when aroused by noxious stimuli but more often only by pain.

Coma is the absence of verbal or complex motor responses to any stimulus (Stevens 2006).

Basic assessments

1. Pupillary functions may be normal if the lesion is rostral to the midbrain, while if the injury is diffuse, e.g., global cerebral anoxia or ischemia, the pupillary abnormality is bilateral. Pupil size is important as midposition (2-5 mm) fixed or irregular pupils imply a focal midbrain lesion; pinpoint reactive pupils occur in global hypoxic ischemic insult with pontine damage, or poisoning with opiates and cholinergic active materials; and bilateral fixed and dilated pupils can reflect central herniation or global hypoxic ischemic or poisoning with barbiturates, scopolamine, and atropine. Unilateral dilated pupil suggests compression of the third cranial nerve and midbrain, which necessitates an immediate search for a potentially correctable abnormality to avoid irreversible injury. In case of post-cardiac arrest coma, if pupils remain nonreactive for more than 6-8 hours after resuscitation, the prognosis for neurological recovery is generally guarded (Stevens 2006).

2. Posturing of the body: decorticate posturing (painful stimuli provoke abnormal flexion of upper limbs) indicates a lesion at the thalamus or cortical damage; decerebrate posturing (the arms and legs extend and pronate in response to pain) denotes that the injury is localized to the midbrain

and upper pons; an injury of the lower brain stem (medulla) leads to flaccid extremities.

3. Ocular reflexes: assessment of the brainstem and cortical functions happen through special reflex tests such as the oculocephalic reflex test (Doll's eyes test), oculovestibular reflex test (cold caloric test), nasal tickle, corneal reflex, and the gag reflex.

4. Vital signs: temperature (rectal is most accurate), blood pressure, heart rate (pulse), respiratory rate, and oxygen saturation (Inouye 2006). It is mandatory to evaluate these basic vital signs quickly and efficiently to gain insight into a patient's metabolism, fluid status, heart function, vascular integrity, and tissue oxygenation status.

5. The respiratory pattern (breathing rhythm) is significant and should be noted in a comatose patient. Certain stereotypical patterns of breathing have been identified including Cheyne- Stokes respiratory pattern, where the patient's breathing is described as alternating episodes of hyperventilation and apnea, a dangerous pattern often seen in pending herniation, extensive cortical lesions, or brainstem damage. Apneustic breathing is characterized by sudden pauses of inspiration and is due to pontine lesion. Ataxic (Biot's) breathing is an irregular chaotic pattern and is due to a lesion of the medulla. The first priority in managing a comatose patient is to stabilize the vital functions, following the ABC rule (Airway, Breathing, and Circulation). Once a person in a coma is stable, assessment of the underlying cause must be done, including imaging (CT scan, CT angiography, magnetic resonance imaging (MRI), magnetic resonance angiography (MRA) and magnetic resonance venography (MRV) if needed) and special studies, e.g., EEG and transcranial Doppler.

Coma is a medical emergency, and attention must first be directed to maintaining the patient's respiration and circulation as previously mentioned using intubation and ventilation, administration of intravenous fluids or blood and other supportive care as needed. Measurement of electrolytes is a commonly performed diagnostic procedure, most often sodium

and potassium; chloride levels are rarely measured except for arterial blood gases (Bateman 2001). Once a patient is stable and no longer in immediate danger, the medical staff should start parallel work, first investigating the patient to find out any underlying pathology of his presenting illness, second, managing the presenting illness symptoms. Infections must be prevented and a balanced nutrition provided. The nursing staff, to guard against pressure ulcers, may move the patient every 2–3 hours from side to side and, depending on the state of consciousness, sometimes to a chair. Physical therapy may also be used to prevent contractures and orthopedic deformities that would limit recovery for those patients who emerge from coma (Wijdicks 2002).

People may emerge from a coma with a combination of physical, intellectual and psychological difficulties that need special attention; recovery usually occurs gradually and some patients acquire more and more ability to respond, others never progress beyond very basic responses. Regaining consciousness is not instant in all comatose patients: in the first days, patients are only awake for a few minutes, the duration of awake time gradually increases, until they regain full consciousness. The coma patient awakens sometimes in a profound state of confusion, not knowing how they got there and sometimes suffering from dysarthria, the inability to articulate speech, and other disabilities. Time is the best general predictor of a chance of recovery: after 4 months of coma caused by brain damage, the chance of partial recovery is less than 15%, and the chance of full recovery is very low (Wijdicks 2002). Coma which lasts seconds to minutes may result in post-traumatic amnesia (PTA) lasting from hours to days; recovery occurs over days to weeks. Coma which lasts hours to days may result in PTA lasting from days to weeks; its recovery occurs over months. Coma which lasts weeks may result in PTA that lasts months; recovery occurs over months.

General Care of the Comatose Patient

1. Airway protection: adequate oxygenation, ventilation and prevention of aspiration are the most important goals; most patients will require endotracheal intubation and frequent orotracheal suctioning.

2. Intravenous hydration: stuporous patients should receive nothing by mouth; use only isotonic fluids in these patients to avoid increasing the size of the cerebral edema or increased intracranial pressure (ICP).

3. Nutrition: enteral feeds via a small bore nasogastric tube.

4. Skin: the patient must be turned every 1-2 hours to prevent pressure sores; an inflatable or foam mattress and protective heel pads may also be beneficial.

5. Eyes: prevent corneal abrasion by taping the eyelids shut or by applying a lubricant.

6. Bowel care: constipation and gastric stress ulcers should be avoided.

7. Bladder care: indwelling urinary catheters are a common source of infection and should be used judiciously; intermittent catheterization every 6 hours when possible.

8. Joint mobility: passive range of motion daily exercises to prevent contractures.

9. Deep venous thrombosis prophylaxis: subcutaneous anticoagulants and external pneumatic compression stockings or both (Upchurch 1995).

To complete this important critical situation, we will discuss two other categories, the permanent vegetative state and locked- in syndrome.

Permanent Vegetative State

Permanent vegetative state (PVS) means an irreversible state of wakefulness without awareness, associated with sleep-wake cycles and preserved brainstem functions. There are no reliable

set of criteria defining and ensuring diagnosis of PVS in infants under 3 months old, apart from anencephalics.

There are three major categories of disease in adults and children that result in PVS, upon which the outcome of PVS depends:

A. In acute traumatic and nontraumatic brain injury, PVS usually evolves within 1 month of injury from a state of eyes- closed coma to a state of wakefulness without awareness with sleep-wake cycles and preserved brainstem functions.

B. Some degenerative and metabolic disorders of the brain (i.e., late stage of dementia of Alzheimer type, end stage of Parkinson disease, and motor neuron disease, pontine myelinolysis, severe uncorrected hypoglycaemic coma) inevitably progress toward an irreversible vegetative state. Patients who are severely impaired but retain some degree of awareness may lapse briefly into a vegetative state from the effects of medication, infection, superimposed illnesses, or decreased fluid and nutritional intake. Such a temporary encephalopathy must be corrected before labeling that patient with the diagnosis of PVS. Consciousness recovery is unlikely if the vegetative state persists for several months.

C. The third cause is severe developmental malformations of the nervous system - the developmental vegetative state is a form of PVS that affects some infants and children with severe congenital malformations of the nervous system. These children do not acquire awareness of self or their environment. This diagnosis can be made at birth only in infants with anencephaly. For children with other severe malformations who appear vegetative at birth, observation for 3 to 6 months is recommended to determine whether these infants acquire awareness. The majority of such infants who are vegetative at birth remain vegetative; those who acquire awareness usually recover only to a severe disability.

Diagnosis

The vegetative state is diagnosed, according to its definition, as being persistent at least for one month. Based upon class II evidence and consensus that reflects a high degree of clinical certainty, the following criteria is standard concerning PVS:

- PVS can be judged to be permanent, at 12 months after traumatic brain injury in adults and children. Special attention to signs of awareness should be devoted to children during the first year after traumatic injury.
- PVS can be judged to be permanent if it lasts more than 3 months, in case of nontraumatic brain injury in both adults and children.
- The chance for recovery, after these periods, is exceedingly low and recovery is almost always to a severe disability.

Management

When a patient has been diagnosed as being in a PVS by a physician skilled in neurological assessment and diagnosis, physicians have the responsibility of discussing with the family or surrogates the probability of the patient's attaining the various stages of recovery or remaining in a PVS:

- Patients in PVS should receive appropriate medical, nursing, or home care to maintain their personal dignity and hygiene.
- Physicians and the family/surrogates must determine appropriate levels of treatment relative to the administration or withdrawal of 1) medications and other commonly ordered treatments; 2) supplemental oxygen and use of antibiotics; 3) complex organ-sustaining treatments such as dialysis; 4) administration of blood products; and 5) artificial hydration and nutrition.

Recovery from PVS can be defined in terms of recovery of consciousness and function. Recovery of consciousness can be confirmed when a patient shows reliable signs of awareness of

self and their environment, reproducible voluntary behavioral responses to visual and auditory stimuli, and interaction with others. Recovery of function occurs when a patient becomes mobile and is able to communicate, learn, and perform adaptive skills and self care and participate in recreational or vocational activities. Using these parameters, recovery of function can be defined with the Glasgow Outcome Scale.

The life span of adults and children in a PVS proves to be reduced; for most PVS patients, life expectancy ranges from 2 to 5 years and survival beyond 10 years is unusual. Once PVS is considered permanent, a "Do not resuscitate (DNR)" order is appropriate which includes no ventilatory or cardiopulmonary resuscitation. The decision to implement a DNR order, however, may be made earlier in the course of the patient's illness if there is an advanced directive or agreement by the appropriate surrogate of the patient and the physicians responsible for the care of the patient (Plum

2007).

Locked-in Syndrome

Locked-in syndrome usually results in quadriparesis and the inability to speak in otherwise cognitively intact individuals. Patients with locked-in syndrome may be able to communicate with others through coded messages by blinking or moving their eyes, which are often not affected by the paralysis. Patients with locked-in syndrome are conscious and aware with no loss of cognitive functions. They sometimes can retain proprioception and sensation throughout their body. Some patients with locked- in syndrome may have the ability to move some muscles of the face, and some or all of the extraocular eye muscles. Patients with locked-in syndrome lack coordination between breathing and voice that restricts them from producing voluntary sounds, even though the vocal cords themselves are not paralyzed. In children, the commonest cause is a stroke of the ventral pons.

Unlike persistent vegetative state, locked-in syndrome is caused by damage of the lower brain and brainstem without damage to

the upper brain (Leon Carrion 2002). Possible causes of locked-in syndrome include: traumatic brain injury, diseases of the circulatory system, overdose of certain drugs, various causes which lead to damage to the nerve cells, particularly destruction of the myelin sheath, e.g., central pontine myelinolysis secondary to rapid correction of hyponatremia and basilar artery (ischemic or hemorrhagic) stroke.

There is neither a standard treatment for locked-in syndrome, nor is there a cure, but stimulation of muscle reflexes with electrodes (NMES) has been known to help patients regain some muscle function. Assistive computer interface technologies in combination with eye tracking may be used to help patients communicate. Direct brain stimulation research developed a technique that allows locked-in patients to communicate via sniffing (Leon Carrion 2002). It is extremely rare for any significant motor function to return and the majority of locked- in syndrome patients do not regain motor control, but devices are available to help patients communicate. 90% die within the first four months after onset. However, some patients continue to live for much longer periods of time (Bateman 2001).

Brain Death

After exclusion of the previous syndromes, and in the absence of brain stem reflexes, brain death in deeply comatose patients should be established through the following criteria:

1. Irreversible coma
2. Absence of brain stem reflexes
3. Absence of spontaneous respiration (Wood 2004)

3. Documentation and Scores

NAbil Kitchener

Medical documentation is important for communication among health care professionals, for research, legal defense, and reimbursement. Neurological scoring systems are used to assess the severity of illness in patients with neurological emergencies, and can be used to monitor the clinical course, to document complications of therapy and to help identify prognostic factors. Two types of scoring systems are commonly used: neurological scoring systems, to quantify neurological deficits, like the Glasgow Coma Scale or the Mini-Mental Status Examination; and functional scoring systems to characterize patients' abilities to perform activities of daily living, used to quantify the functional outcome with or without therapy, like the Canadian Neurological Score, the NIH stroke scale, the modified Rankin scale, the expanded disability status scale, the Richmond agitation sedation score and the confusion assessment method.
Neurological scoring is used in the critical care unit while scores for activities of daily living are used for the outcome assessment.

Intensive care units (ICUs) provide a service for patients with potentially recoverable diseases who can benefit from more detailed observation and treatment than is usually available on the general wards. Patients may be discharged from the ICU when their physiologic status has stabilized and the need for ICU monitoring and care is no longer necessary

(Egol 1999). However, a number of patients who are successfully discharged from intensive care subsequently die during their hospital admissions. This may indicate premature discharge from the ICU or suboptimal management in the ICU or the general ward (Campbell 2008). As trends move towards earlier ICU discharge, it becomes increasingly important to be able to identify those patients at high risk of subsequent clinical deterioration, who might benefit from longer ICU stays or from transfers to intermediate care units. A strategy to reduce premature discharges in patients at high risk of in-hospital death could result in a 39% reduction in post-ICU death in these patients (Daly 2001). It can be concluded that reliable baseline and follow- up assessment is crucial to document any improvement or deterioration in neurological status of patients admitted to a neurocritical care unit. Interrater differences may be significant, so the need for standardized neurological scales and scores comes into play.

Scales seek to quantify different aspects of function within the framework of the World Health Organization hierarchy of impairment, disability, and handicap (Thuriaux 1995). Since the introduction of the Mathew scale in 1972 (Mathew 1972), there has been a steadily increasing number of scales that seek to quantify neurological impairment. These scales involve scoring different modalities of neurological function and then sum the scores to provide an index for neurological status. These scales were developed for a variety of reasons, including monitoring neurological status for improvement or deterioration (Cote 1986) and predicting final outcome in a defined group of patients (Brott 1989). The primary purpose for these scales in neurocritical care units is to compare the baseline neurological impairment severity of patients at admission, and to quantify neurological recovery over time, to avoid premature discharge from the neurocritical care unit and promote early detection of deterioration and prompt management.

Scoring and Documentation

Each neurocritical care unit should adopt a special scoring and documentation system, to be used to assess and document baseline patient neurological status and status at time of discharge. These include:
- Vital Signs: BP, temp, pulse, respiration, oximetry
- Pupils: size and reaction to light
- Eye movement: gaze, vergence, individual extraocular movement and nystagmus
- Mental status: LOC, orientation and speech
- Motor functions: state, power, tone, deep reflexes and pathological reflexes
- Coordination: gate, upper and lower limbs, if applicable

There are many scales used to assess these functions; each critical care unit can adopt a set that can be used by its staff. Tables 3.1, 3.2, and 3.3 show some of the commonly used scales in clinical practice.

Table 3.1 – Neurological Scales used for assessment of level of consciousness and mental status

Name and Source	Strengths and Weaknesses
Level-of-consciousness scale	
Glasgow Coma Scale (Teasdale 1974, 1979)	Strength: Simple, valid, reliable, for assessment of level-of-consciousness. Weaknesses: none observed.
Full Outline Unresponsiveness – FOUR Score (Wijdicks 2005)	Strength: The FOUR score is easy to apply and provides more neurological details than the Glasgow scale. This scale is able to detect conditions such locked-in syndrome and the vegetative state, which are not detected by the GCS. Weaknesses: none observed.
Delirium Scale	
Confusion Assessment Method (CAM) (Inouye 1990)	Strength: CAM-ICU is an adaptation of the Confusion Assessment Method (CAM), which was adapted to be a delirium assessment tool for use in ICU patients (e.g., critically ill patients on and off the ventilator who are largely unable to talk). Weaknesses: none observed.
Richmond Agitation Sedation Scale (RASS) (Sessler 2002)	Strength: RASS is logical, easy to administer, and readily recalled. RASS has high reliability and validity in medical and surgical, ventilated and non-ventilated, and sedated and non-sedated adult ICU patients. Weaknesses: none observed
Mental status screening	
Folstein Mini-Mental State Examination (Folstein 1975)	Strength: Widely used for screening. Weaknesses: Several functions with summed score. May mis-classify patients with aphasia.
Neurobehavioral Cognition Status Exam (NCSE) (Kiernan 1987)	Strength: Predicts gain in Barthel Index scores. Unrelated to age. Weaknesses: Does not distinguish right from left hemisphere. No reliability studies in stroke. No studies of factorial structure. Correlates with education.

Table 3.2 – Neurological Scales used for assessment of stroke deficits

Name and Source	Strengths	Weaknesses
Measures of disability/activities of daily living (ADL)		
Barthel Index (Mahoney 1965, Wade 1988)	Widely used for stroke. Excellent validity and reliability.	Low sensitivity for high-level functioning
Functional Independence Measure (FIM) (Granger 1987)	Widely used for stroke. Measures mobility, ADL, cognition, functional communication.	"Ceiling" and "floor" effects
Stroke deficit scales		
NIH Stroke Scale (Brott 1989)	Brief, reliable, can be administered by non-neurologists	Low sensitivity
Canadian Neurological Scale (Cote 1986)	Brief, valid, reliable	Some useful measures omitted
Assessment of motor function		
Fugl-Meyer (Fugl-Meyer 1975)	Extensively evaluated measure. Good validity and reliability for assessing sensorimotor function and balance	Considered too complex and time-consuming by many
Motor Assessment Scale (Poole 1988)	Good, brief assessment of movement and physical mobility	Reliability assessed only in stable patients. Sensitivity not tested
Motricity Index (Collin 1990)	Brief assessment of motor function of arm, leg, and trunk	Sensitivity not tested
Balance assessment		
Berg Balance Assessment (Berg 1992)	Simple, well established with stroke patients, sensitive to change	None observed
Mobility assessment		
Rivermead Mobility Index (Collen 1991)	Valid, brief, reliable test of physical mobility	Sensitivity not tested

Name and Source	Strengths	Weaknesses
Assessment of speech and language functions		
Boston Diagnostic Aphasia Examination (Goodglass 1983)	Widely used, comprehensive, good standardization data, sound theoretical rationale	Long time to administer; half of patients cannot be classified
Porch Index of Communicative Ability (PICA) (Porch 1981)	Widely used, comprehensive, careful test development and standardization	Long time to administer. Special training required to administer. Inadequate sampling of language other than one word and single sentences
Western aphasia Battery (Kertesz 1982)	Widely used, comprehensive	Long time to administer. "Aphasia quotients" and "taxonomy" of aphasia not well validated

Table 3.3 – Neurological Scales used for assessment of health status and global disabilities

Type	Name and Source	Strengths	Weaknesses
Global disability scale	Rankin Scale (Rankin 1957, Bonita 1988, Van Swieten 1988)	Good for overall assessment of disability.	Walking is the only explicit assessment criterion. Low sensitivity
Health status/quality of life measures	Medical Outcomes Study (MOS) 36 Item Short-Form Health Survey (Ware 1992)	Generic health status scale SF36 is improved version of SF20. Brief, can be self-administered or administered by phone or interview. Widely used in the US	Possible "floor" effect in seriously ill patients (especially for physical functioning), suggests it should be supplemented by an ADL scale in stroke patients
	Sickness Impact Profile (SIP) (Bergner 1981)	Comprehensive and well-evaluated. Broad range of items reduces "floor" or "ceiling" effects	Time to administer somewhat long. Evaluates behavior rather than subjective health; needs questions on well-being, happiness, and satisfaction

Delirium

Delirium is a disturbance of consciousness characterized by acute onset and fluctuating course of inattention accompanied by either a change in cognition or a perceptual disturbance, so that a patient's ability to receive, process, store, and recall information is impaired.

Delirium, a medical emergency, develops rapidly over a short period of time, is usually reversible, and is a direct consequence of a medical condition or a brain insult. Many delirious ICU patients have recently been comatose, indicating a fluctuation of mental status. Comatose patients often, but not always, progress through a period of delirium before recovering to their baseline mental status.

ICU delirium is a predictor of increased mortality, length of stay, time on ventilator, costs, re-intubation, long-term cognitive impairment, and discharge to long-term care facility; it necessitates special attention, assessment and management.

Delirium assessment is actually an important part of the overall assessment of consciousness.

Delirium includes three subtypes: hyperactive, hypoactive and mixed. Hyperactive delirium is characterized by agitation, restlessness, and attempts to remove tubes and lines. Hypoactive delirium is characterized by withdrawal, flat affect, apathy, lethargy, and decreased responsiveness. Mixed delirium is characterized by fluctuation between the hypoactive and hyperactive. In ICU patients mixed and hypoactive are the most common, and are often undiagnosed if routine monitoring is not implemented. Few ICU patients (less than 5%) experience purely hyperactive delirium.

The Confusion Assessment Method (CAM) was created in 1990 by Sharon Inouye, and was intended to be a bedside assessment tool usable by non-psychiatrists to assess for delirium (Inouye 1990). The CAM-ICU is an adaptation of this tool for use in ICU patients (e.g., critically ill patients on and off the ventilator who are largely unable to talk).

4. Brain Injuries

MAgdy KhAlAf, NAbil Kitchener

Neurocritical care focuses on critically ill patients with primary or secondary neurological problems. Initially neurocritical care was developed to manage postoperative neurosurgical patients; it then expanded to the management of patients with traumatic brain injury (TBI), intracranial hemorrhage and complications of subarachnoid hemorrhage, including vasospasm, elevated intracranial pressure (ICP) and the cardiopulmonary complications of brain injury (Bamford 1992). The striking improvements noted in many studies suggest that high-quality neurocritical care with the delivery of targeted therapeutic interventions does have an impact, not only on survival, but importantly also on the quality of survival.

Types of Brain Injuries

Primary brain injuries

Ischemic brain injury: either global, which includes cardiac arrest or anoxia, or regional ischemic brain injury, which includes vasospasm, compression of blood vessels or stroke. Stroke can be classified into ischemic and hemorrhagic strokes.

Ischemic stroke accounts for 80% of all strokes and can be further classified into thrombotic or embolic stroke; ischemic thrombotic stroke accounts for 77% while ischemic embolic stroke constitutes the remainder.

Hemorrhagic strokes constitute 10-20% of all strokes, and can be further classified into two types, the intracerebral hemorrhage that constitutes up to 75% and the subarachnoid hemorrhage that makes up the other 25%.

Acute ischemic stroke is the third leading cause of death in industrialized countries and the most frequent cause of permanent disability in adults worldwide, so understanding the pathogenesis of ischemic stroke is mandatory. Despite great strides in understanding the pathophysiology of cerebral ischemia, therapeutic options remain limited. Only recombinant tissue plasminogen activator (rTPA) for thrombolysis is currently approved for use in the management of acute ischemic stroke.

However, its use is limited by its short therapeutic window (3-4.5 hours), complications from the risk of hemorrhage, and the potential damage from reperfusion injury. Effective stroke management requires recanalization of the occluded blood vessels. However, reperfusion can cause neurovascular injury, leading to cerebral edema, brain hemorrhage, and neuronal death by apoptosis or necrosis (Hajjar 2011).

Central nervous system (CNS) infections: Acute onset fever with altered mental status is a problem commonly encountered by the physician in the emergency setting. "Acute febrile encephalopathy" is a commonly used term for description of the altered mental status that either accompanies or follows a short febrile illness. CNS infections are the most common cause of nontraumatic disturbed consciousness. The etiologic agents may be viruses, bacteria, or parasites. Central nervous system infections are classified into categories beginning with those in immunocompetent hosts followed by infection with the human immunodeficiency virus (HIV) and its opportunistic infections. The viruses responsible for most cases of acute encephalitis in immunocompetent hosts are herpes viruses, arboviruses, and enteroviruses. Neurotropic herpes viruses that cause

encephalitis predominantly in immunocompetent hosts include herpes simplex virus 1 (HSV-1) and 2 (HSV-2), human herpes virus 6 (HHV-6) and 7 (HHV-7), and Epstein-Barr virus (EBV).
Cytomegalovirus (CMV) and varicella-zoster virus (VZV) may in some situations cause encephalitis in immunocompetent patients, but more commonly they produce an opportunistic infection in immunocompromised individuals, such as those with HIV infection, organ transplant recipients, or other patients using immunosuppressive drugs. HSV-1 is the most common cause of severe sporadic viral encephalitis in the United States; diagnosis has been become more familiar due to the availability of cerebrospinal fluid (CSF) polymerase chain reaction (PCR) analysis techniques that allow for rapid, specific, and sensitive diagnoses. The use of CSF PCR instead of brain biopsy as the diagnostic standard for HSV encephalitis has expanded awareness of mild or atypical cases of HSV encephalitis. Adult encephalitis is caused by 2 viral serotypes, HSV-1 and HSV-2.
Patients with greater than 100 DNA copies/μL HSV in CSF are more likely than those with fewer copies to have a reduced level of consciousness, more significant abnormal findings on neuroimaging, a longer duration of illness, higher mortality, and more sequelae (Domingues 1997). EBV is almost never cultured from CSF during infection, and serological testing is inconclusive, so CSF PCR diagnosis is mandatory.
Semiquantitative PCR analysis of EBV DNA suggests that copy numbers are significantly higher in patients with active EBV infection. HHV-6 and -7 can cause exanthema subitum, and appear to be associated with febrile convulsions, even in

the absence of signs of exanthema subitum. Almost all children (>90%) with exanthema subitum have HHV-6 or HHV-7 DNA in CSF. Inflammatory primary brain damage like meningitis and encephalitis come from pyogenic infections that reach the intracranial structures in one of two ways - either by hematogenous spread (infected thrombi or emboli of bacteria) or by extension from cranial structures (ears, paranasal sinuses, osteomyelitic foci in the skull, penetrating cranial injuries or congenital sinus tracts). In a good number of cases, infection is iatrogenic, being introduced in the course of cerebral or spinal surgery, during the placement of a ventriculoperitoneal shunt or rarely through a lumbar puncture needle. Nowadays, nosocomial infections are as frequent as the non-hospital acquired variety. The reason for altered sensorium in meningitis is postulated to be the spillage of inflammatory cells to the adjacent brain parenchyma and the resultant brain edema (Levin 1998).

Compressive brain injury: e.g., tumors and cerebral brain edema are considered as important causes for impairment of the level of consciousness. During tumor growth, cerebral tissues adjacent to the tumor and nearby venules are compressed, which results in elevation of capillary pressure, particularly in the cerebral white matter, and there is a change in cerebral blood flow and consequently intracranial pressure. At that stage the tumor begins to displace tissue, which eventually leads to displacement of tissue at a distance from the tumor, resulting in false localizing signs such as transtentorial herniations, paradoxical corticospinal signs of Kernohan and Woltman, third and sixth nerve palsies and secondary hydrocephalus, originally described in tumor patients.

Secondary brain injuries

Secondary brain injuries include renal coma, hepatic coma, salt and water imbalance, disturbance of glucose metabolism, other endocrinal causes of coma, disturbances of calcium and magnesium metabolism, drug intoxication and other material intoxication, not only drug toxicity, hypertensive and metabolic encephalopathies, sleep apnea syndromes and other ventilator disturbances. Mechanisms of secondary brain injury include hypoxia, hypoperfusion, reperfusion injury with free radical formations, release of excitatory amino acids and harmful mediators from injured cells, electrolyte and acid base changes from systemic or regional ischemia (Semplicini 2003).

The primary goal in managing neurologically compromised patients includes (Stasiukyniene 2009) stabilizing the brain

through the maintenance of oxygen delivery via the

following parameters:
1. Assuring systemic oxygen transport and adequate oxygenation, maintaining hemoglobin level (at approximately 10 g/dl or more) and cardiac output.
2. Assuring optimal mean arterial pressure (MAP). Many insults are associated with hypertension, which may be a physiologic compensation, so excessive lowering of blood pressure may induce secondary ischemia. In general, systolic pressure should be treated when more than 200 mmHg or MAP when more than 125 mmHg. Cautious reduction in mean arterial pressure by only 25% is recommended (Adams 2007).
3. Avoiding prophylactic or routine hyperventilation - a decrease in extracellular brain pH may produce vasoconstriction in responsive vessels and reduce CBF to already ischemic zones. This applies to patients with head trauma in whom routine hyperventilation is no longer considered desirable; brief hyperventilation may be lifesaving in the patient with herniation,

pending the institution of other methods to lower elevated ICP.
4. Assuring euvolemia. Hypervolemia may also be helpful when vasoconstriction is suspected, as in the setting of subarachnoid hemorrhage.
5. Consideration should be given to administering intravenous lidocaine 1.5 mg/kg or intravenous thiopental (5 mg/kg) to blunt the rise in ICP associated with intubation.
6. Nimodipine should be instituted immediately in patients with SAH and is advocated by some in patients with subarachnoid bleeding after head trauma. Nimodipine probably improves outcome by decreasing calcium-mediated neuronal toxicity.
7. Using normal saline as the primary maintenance fluid; dextrose administration is usually avoided unless the patient is hypoglycemic; hypotonic solutions should also be avoided.
8. Assessing and treating coagulation defects.
9. Sedation and/or neuromuscular blockade after intubation may be required to control harmful agitation.
10. If seizure occurrs, it should be aggressively treated.
11. Titration of the ICP and cerebral perfusion pressure.

Management of Special Issues
Traumatic brain injury

Outcome after traumatic brain injury depends upon the initial severity of the injury, age, the extent of any subsequent complications, and how these are managed. Much of the early management of traumatic brain injury falls upon emergency room staff, primary care and ambulance services prior to hospital admission. Most patients who attend hospital after a traumatic brain injury do not develop life-threatening complications in the acute stage. However, in a small but important subgroup, the outcome is made worse by failure to detect promptly and deal adequately with complications.

General rules:
1. A traumatic brain injury should be discussed with neurosurgery when
   a. a CT scan in a general hospital shows a recent intracranial lesion
   b. a patient fulfills the criteria for CT scanning but this cannot be done within an appropriate period
   c. whatever the result of the CT scan, the patient has clinical features that suggest that specialist neurological assessment, monitoring, or management are appropriate. Reasons include:
      i. Persistent coma (GCS <9, no eye opening) after initial resuscitation
      ii. Confusion persisting for more than 4 hours
      iii. Deterioration in level of consciousness after admission (a sustained decrease of one point in the motor or verbal GCS subscores, or 2 points on the eye opening subscale of the GCS)
      iv. Persistent focal neurological signs
      v. A seizure without full recovery
      vi. Compound depressed fracture
      vii. Suspected or definite penetrating injury
      viii. A CSF leak or other sign of base of skull fracture
2. Keep sodium >140 mmol/L. A fall in serum sodium produces an osmotic gradient across the blood–brain barrier, and aggravates cerebral edema.
3. Avoid hyperglycemia (treat blood glucose >11 mmol/L). Hyperglycemia increases cerebral lactic acidosis, which may aggravate ischemic brain injury.
4. Feed via an orogastric tube. Gastric motility agents can be given as required.

5. Use TED stockings; avoid low-dose heparin.
6. Apply 15–30° head-up tilt with head kept in neutral position; this may improve CPP.
7. No parenteral hypotonic fluid must be given.

Acute stroke

The World Stroke Organization declared a public health emergency on World Stroke Day (WSO 2010). There are 15 million people who have a stroke each year. According to the World Health Organization, stroke is the second leading cause of death for people above the age of 60, and the fifth leading cause in people aged 15 to 59. Stroke also happens to children, including newborns. Each year, nearly six million people die from stroke. In fact, stroke is responsible for more deaths annually than those attributed to AIDS, tuberculosis and malaria put together. Stroke is also the leading cause of long-term disability irrespective of age, gender, ethnicity or country.

Yet for many healthcare staff it remains an area of therapeutic nihilism and thus uninteresting and neglected (WSO 2010). This

negative perception is shared by the general public, who often has a poor understanding of the early symptoms and significance of a stroke.

Yet within the last few years there have been many important developments in the approach to awareness and caring for stroke patients, for both the acute management and secondary prevention. Clinical research and interest in stroke has increased greatly in the last few years. Each minute of brain ischemia causes the destruction of 1.9 million neurons, 14 billion synapses, and 7.5 miles of myelinated nerves (Hand 2006).

Ischemic stroke is characterized by one or more focal neurological deficits corresponding to the ischemic brain regions. It requires an immediate decision regarding thrombolytic therapy (tissue plasminogen activator, TPA, in the dosage of 0.9 mg/kg, 10% as a bolus over 1 minute and infuse the remaining 90% over the next hour).

Wise control of hypertension is essential, control of hyperglycemia and fever is protective against more destruction of neurons (Mistri 2006).

Status epilepticus (SE)

Status epilepticus is defined as more than 30 minutes of continuous seizure activity or recurrent seizure activity without an intervening period of consciousness (Manno 2003).

In one survey, only 10% of patients who develop seizures in a medical ICU will develop SE. The most common causes of SE are noncompliance with or withdrawal of antiepileptic medications, cerebrovascular disease and alcohol withdrawal.

The hypersynchronous neuronal discharge that characterizes a seizure is mediated by an imbalance between excitation and inhibition. The adverse effects of generalized seizures include hypertension, lactic acidosis, hyperthermia, respiratory compromise, pulmonary aspiration or edema, rhabdomyolysis, self-injury and irreversible neurological damage (Bassin 2002).

The most common and potentially dangerous forms of status epilepticus are generalized convulsive status epilepticus, non-

convulsive generalized status epilepticus, refractory status epilepticus and myoclonic status epilepticus. Also, seizures that persist for longer than 5-10 minutes should be treated urgently because of the risk of permanent neurological injury and because seizures become refractory to therapy the longer they persist (Stasiukyniene 2009).

General measures for management are shown in Table 4.1.

Intravenous drug therapy for convulsive seizures in the ICU are as follows:

1. Lorazepam: 0.10 mg/kg up to 2 mg/min or diazepam 0.15 mg/kg; if seizure continues, give

2. Fosphenytoin: 20 mg/kg up to 150 mg/min or phenytoin 20 mg/kg up to 50 mg/min; if seizure continues, one of the following medications may be used but these require intubation and mechanical ventilation:
   - phenobarbital 20 mg/kg up to 50 mg/min
   - propofol 3-5 mg/kg load then 1-15 mg/kg/hr
   - midazolam 0.2 mg/kg load then 0.05-2 mg/kg/hr
   - pentobarbital 5-15 mg/kg load, then 0.5-10 mg/kg/hr

Neuromuscular emergencies

Neuromuscular emergencies are composed of a group of severe life-threatening neuromuscular diseases such as myasthenic crises, cholinergic crises, critical illness myopathy and critical illness polyneuropathy.

Respiratory paralysis occurs in a small percentage of patients with acute neuromuscular disease and accounts for less than 1% of admissions to general intensive care units. Its development may be insidious so that patients with acute neuromuscular disease should have their vital capacity monitored. Orotracheal intubation and ventilatory support should be instituted prophylactically when vital capacity is falling towards 15 ml/kg. Earlier intervention is necessary in the presence of bulbar palsy.

Table 4.1 – General measures for management of Status Epilepticus*

1 (0–10 minutes)
Assess cardiorespiratory function
Secure airway and resuscitate
Administer oxygen
2 (0–60 minutes)
Institute regular monitoring
Emergency antiepileptic drug therapy Set up intravenous lines
Emergency investigations
Administer glucose (50 ml of 50% solution) and/or intravenous thiamine (250 mg) as high potency intravenous Pabrinex where appropriate Treat acidosis if severe
3 (0–60/90 minutes)
Establish etiology
Identify and treat medical complications Pressor therapy where appropriate
4 (30–90 minutes)
Transfer to intensive care
Establish intensive care and EEG monitoring Initiate seizure and EEG monitoring
Initiate intracranial pressure monitoring where appropriate Initiate long term, maintenance, antiepileptic therapy
These four stages should be followed chronologically; the first and second within 10 minutes, and stage 4 (transfer to intensive care unit) in most settings within 60–90 minutes of presentation.

*Derived from Shorvon 1994

After assessment of these important conditions, and once the respiratory consequences of progressive neuromuscular weakness are established, the following requirements for management of critical neuromuscular diseases in ICU should be fulfilled:

1. Continuous monitoring of oxygen saturation to stay above 95%; pacemaker to be considered if heart rate variability is abnormal.
2. Assessment of muscle strength through measurement

of vital capacity, hand grip strength (dynamometer), arm abduction time, head lifting time, loudness of voice, ability to swallow secretions and use of accessory muscles of ventilation.

3. Management of inability to swallow through frequent suction, head positioning to allow use of a nasogastric, an orogastric or a Guedel tube.
4. Assessment of cardiac output, e.g., in myositis and arrhythmias (autonomic fiber involvement in GBS), heparinization for prevention of deep venous thrombosis, care for decubital ulcers.
5. Indications for intubation and artificial ventilation in neuromuscular critical cases: If oxygen saturation is below 90% (below 85% if more chronic), exhaustive respiratory work, forced vital capacity falling below 15 ml/kg and recurrent minor aspiration, avoid use of muscle relaxants. If artificial ventilation is likely to be required for more than approx. seven days, a tracheostomy should be created and is more comfortable for the patient than continued orotracheal intubation. Nutrition should be provided early via a nasogastric tube. Strenuous efforts should be made to reduce the incidence of nosocomial infection. Patients with neuropathy should be monitored for autonomic dysfunction causing cardiac arrhythmia or fluctuating blood pressure. Deep vein thrombosis should be avoided by regular passive limb movements and low-dose subcutaneous heparin.
6. Use assisted ventilation with IMV mode with low PEEP of 3 cm H_2O except in pneumonia, atelectasis and use as few sedatives as possible to monitor neurologic findings (Murray 2002). Critical illness polyneuropathy and myopathy are considered conditions associated with inflammatory injury to

major organs involving peripheral nerves and skeletal muscles, and may add considerable value to the morbidity and mortality of the ICU stays.

7. If systolic pressure remains below 90 mmHg after adequate volume replacement, begin dopamine infusion to maintain systolic pressure above 90 mmHg; if dopamine is inadequate maintain dopamine and start dobutamine infusion. If the patient develops diabetes insipidus with

urine output exceeding 250 ml/hour for 2 hours, start a vasopressin infusion at a dose of 0.5-1.0 U/hour for adults, titrate infusion to maintain urine output at 100-200 ml/hour. Send tracheal aspirate, urine and blood for routine and fungal culture (Shoemaker 2000).

Metabolic disturbances such as hypokalemia or hypermagnesemia should always be looked for and corrected first. In Guillain–Barré syndrome we recommend intravenous immunoglobulin as being equally effective to plasma exchange, safer, and more convenient. In myasthenia gravis we recommend intravenous immunoglobulin followed by thymectomy or, where thymectomy is inappropriate or has been unsuccessful, intravenous immunoglobulin combined with azathioprine and steroids. In polymyositis and dermatomyositis, steroids are the mainstay of treatment but intravenous immunoglobulin is also effective.

Management of subarachnoid hemorrhage

Subarachnoid hemorrhage (SAH) is a complex medical and surgical event. Among its multiple etiologies, one of the most common relates to bleeding from a cerebral aneurysm. The optimal management of this life-threatening condition relies on a systematic and organized approach leading to the correct diagnosis and timely referral to a capable neurosurgeon. The following is a brief summary of steps that should be initiated when SAH is suspected, and the role of a medical neurocritical care facility.

A CT scan should be obtained immediately after the diagnosis is suspected. If the CT scan is positive, lumbar puncture is unnecessary and even dangerous due to the risks of aneurismal rebleeding or transtentorial brain herniation. If the CT scan is negative, lumbar puncture may be helpful if the history of the ictal headache is not typical of subarachnoid hemorrhage, insidious in onset, or of migrainous character. If the patient relates a history typical of SAH, a cerebral CT arteriogram should be performed despite a negative CT scan. Up to 15% of CT scans obtained within 48 hours of SAH will be negative.

Once the diagnosis is confirmed with a CT scan, a neurosurgeon who can treat the patient should be contacted immediately.

Delays in transfer may prove fatal because of the potential for aneurismal rebleeding prior to intervention. It is often best to allow the interventionist or surgeon who will be caring for the patient to arrange for the diagnostic arteriogram to be performed at the institution where the patient will undergo intervention or surgery to repair the aneurysm. Arteriography performed by institutions infrequently treating SAH may be technically inadequate and require repetition upon transfer to the interventionist.

Blood pressure must be closely monitored and controlled following SAH. Hypertension will increase the chance of catastrophic rebleeding. Blood pressure control should be initiated immediately upon diagnosis of SAH.

Medical preoperative management includes prophylactic anticonvulsants, calcium channel blockade, corticosteroids, and antihypertensives as needed. We do not initiate antifibrinolytic therapy unless surgery is not considered within 48 hours of the initial SAH.

Medications that can be initiated prior to transfer to interventionist or neurosurgeon include:
- dexamethasone, 4 mg IV six hourly
- nimodipine, 60 mg orally four hourly
- phenytoin, 10 mg/kg IV load, then 100 mg orally/IV three times daily

A frequent source of diagnostic difficulty for the interventionist lies in the use of excessive amounts of narcotic analgesics prior to transfer to the neurosurgical service.

Although pain control facilitates blood pressure control, the ability to grade accurately the patient's level of consciousness has significant impact on the timing of intervention. Clinical

grading also, obscured by large doses of narcotic analgesics, makes surgical planning more difficult.

5. Basic Hemodynamic Monitoring of Neurocritical Patients

BAssem ZArif, MAgdy KhAlAf, NAbil Kitchener

The importance of basic hemodynamic monitoring of neurocritical patients comes from the goal of maintaining brain autoregulation. Brain autoregulation and other biological signals are the variables to be monitored by using biomedical sensors.

Complications that may occur in neurocritical patients (e.g., sepsis, dehydration, post-cardiac arrest status) make hemodynamic monitoring of greater importance.

The goals of hemodynamic monitoring in neurocritical care units are to assess the magnitude of physiological derangements in critically ill patients and to institute measures to correct the imbalance.

The following steps should be taken to reach these goals. Although our review of data may be helpful, the attending physician should decide what to use and when to use it. Menu to work with for proper patient management:

1. Pulse oximeter (SpO_2) is regarded as one of the most important advances in critical care monitoring. SpO_2 provides a continuous non-invasive method to measure arterial oxygen saturation, and should be used on every neurocritical patient. The absorption spectra of both oxyhemoglobin and deoxyhemoglobin and the characteristics of pulsatile blood can thus be determined. SpO_2 is

accurate to within ± 2% for saturations >70%. SpO_2 is widely used in monitoring patients who have a variety of neurological conditions (Adams 1997), and calculations made from the processed signals provide estimates of the tissue or venous and arterial blood and provide an estimate of the amount of oxygenated hemoglobin and the percent saturation of hemoglobin by oxygen SaO_2, which is not the same as the PaO_2 (partial pressure of oxygen) in the blood (Adams 1997). The PaO_2 and SaO_2 measurements of oxygenation are related through the oxyhemoglobin dissociation curve. Importantly, SpO_2 is a measure of arterial oxygenation saturation, not arterial oxygen tension (PaO_2). Given the characteristics of the oxygen dissociation curve, large fluctuations in PaO_2 can occur despite minimal changes in SpO_2. In addition to its inability to measure PaO_2, SpO_2 provides no measure of ventilation or acid-base status. Therefore, it cannot be used to determine pH or arterial carbon dioxide tension. Significant increases in arterial carbon dioxide can occur with normal readings in SpO_2.

Although useful for arterial oxygen saturation, SpO_2 should not be assumed to provide information about ventilation. Studies have shown that to assure a saturation of 60 torr (8.0 kPa), an SpO_2 of 92% should be maintained in patients with light skin, whereas 94% saturation may be needed in patients with dark skin. Oxygenation is considered adequate if the arterial oxygen saturation is above 95%. The majority of these patients are placed on positive end expiratory pressure

(PEEP) at 5cm H_2O (Curley 1990).

Also, for patients with manifestations consistent with hypoxemia (e.g., tachycardia, hypotension, anxiety, and agitation) there is a time delay in pulse oximeter to express fluctuation in SpO_2. Again in hypothermia, low CO_2, and vasoconstriction secondary to drugs or peripheral hypoxia

all increase bias, imprecision, and response time for hypoxic episodes, so we proceed to the next step.
2. Arterial blood gas analysis is widely available in hospitals and offers direct measurements of many critical parameters (pH, PaO_2, $PaCO_2$). Arterial blood gas analysis is among the most precise measurements of oxygen tension and pressure that will reflect tissue oxygenation (García 2011).
3. Non-invasive automated blood pressure devices are frequently used to obtain non-invasive, intermittent blood pressure measurements. Measurements of systolic and diastolic pressure to calculate the mean arterial pressure (MAP) is mandatory to calculate the cerebral perfusion pressure. These devices are less accurate in critically ill patients as well as in those with secondary brain injury. These less accurate readings can distract the attention of the caregiver. The evaluation of blood pressure will be significantly affected by the use of vasopressors. Therefore, the numeric reading may reflect vasoconstriction in spite of decreasing perfusion with adequate blood pressure.
4. Invasive blood pressure monitoring for continuous monitoring and recording of the arterial pressure via an arterial catheter is preferable to the use of an automated blood pressure device in hemodynamically unstable patients (García 2011). The radial artery is most commonly cannulated because of its superficial

location, relative ease of cannulation, and in most patients, adequate collateral flow from the ulnar artery. Other potential sites for percutaneous arterial cannulation include the femoral, brachial, axillary, ulnar, dorsalis pedis, and posterior tibial arteries. Possible complications of intra-arterial monitoring include hematoma, neurologic injury, arterial embolization, limb ischemia, infection, and inadvertent intra-arterial injection of drugs. Intra-arterial catheters are not placed in extremities with potential vascular insufficiency. However, with proper selection, the complication rate associated with intra-arterial cannulation is low and the benefits can be important.

5. A Foley catheter, for monitoring of urine output on an hourly basis or for 24 hours, is a simple and important tool to monitor volume status of the patient besides renal perfusion and function. The hourly urine output is a cheap, simple and indirect method of assessing adequacy of cardiac output and tissue perfusion.

6. A temperature probe is also indicated for purposes of monitoring core temperature.

7. Continuous monitoring of volume status and other parameters:

    If the patient is hypotensive, a fluid supplement with 1-2 liters Ringer's lactate for 30-60 minutes is reasonable.

    Subsequent fluid management should be based upon urine output and maintaining central venous pressure between 5 and 10 mmHg. Monitor potassium, sodium, glucose and arterial blood gases every 4 hours. Especially if there is respiratory embarrassment at initial evaluation, measurement of hematocrit, magnesium, blood urea nitrogen, creatinine, calcium, liver function tests, urine analysis, prothrombin, partial thromboplastin times and phosphate levels are mandatory. If hematocrit is below 30%, transfuse cross-matched blood (Amin 1993).

8. Common indications for central venous cannulation: measurement of mean central venous pressure, large bore venous access, administration of irritating drugs and or parenteral nutrition, hemodialysis, placement of a pulmonary artery catheter.

Placement of a pulmonary artery catheter is indicated to obtain direct and calculated hemodynamic data that cannot be obtained through less invasive means (Sakr 2005).

The goal for all critically ill patients is to provide adequate oxygen for cellular use through suitable oxygen consumption, which is variable between tissues, and the changes of the basal or active metabolic rate for each cell.

Oxygen delivery to tissues and organs responds to many local systemic variables to keep cellular homeostasis.

Pulmonary artery balloon flotation catheter insertion may be necessary for full assessment of these parameters, and of evaluation of determinants of cardiac output and the oxygen content of circulating blood, on which oxygen delivery is dependent. In the presence of positive pressure ventilation with PEEP, central venous and pulmonary artery occlusion pressures may be falsely elevated and need to be interpreted with caution. The fluid challenge is the only way to interpret Central Venous Pressure (CVP) or Pulmonary Artery Occlusion Pressure (PAOP).

Assessment of the determinants of cardiac output will proceed as follows:

a. Heart rate and rhythm assisted by pulse oximeter and electrocardiogram.

b. Preload assessed right and left heart; right heart through neck vein distension, liver enlargement and central venous pressure assessment; left heart through dyspnea on exertion, orthopnea, arterial blood pressure; pulmonary artery occlusion pressure and arterial pressure through waveform analysis (Sakr 2005).
c. Afterload assisted by mean arterial blood pressure and systemic vascular resistance; contractility can be assessed by ejection fraction and echocardiography.

As discussed earlier, the goal of hemodynamic monitoring in neurocritical care units is to assess the magnitude of physiological derangements in critically ill patients and to institute measures to correct the imbalance. Basic hemodynamic monitoring consists of clinical examination, invasive arterial monitoring, central venous pressure monitoring, hourly urine output, central venous oxygen saturation and echocardiography. Dynamic indices of fluid responsiveness such as the pulse pressure variation and stroke volume variation can guide decision making for fluid resuscitation. Cardiac output is traditionally measured using the pulmonary artery catheter; less invasive methods now available include the pulse contour analysis and arterial pulse pressure derived methods. It is essential to determine whether the hemodynamic therapy is resulting in an adequate supply of oxygen to the tissues proportionate to their demand. Mixed and central venous oxygen saturation and lactate levels are commonly used to determine the balance between oxygen supply and demand (Walley 2011).

6. Neurocritical Monitoring
MervAt WAhbA, NAbil Kitchener, Simin MAnsoor

Neurocritical care relies on monitoring cerebral functions. Intracranial pressure monitoring may indicate high pressure in several acute neurological conditions. Massive stroke may cause life-threatening brain edema and occur in about 10% of patients with supratentorial stroke. Massive brain edema usually occurs between the second and the fifth day after stroke onset. Case fatality rates may exceed 80%. Other neurologic conditions that may be accompanied with increased intracranial pressure include severe head injuries, status epilepticus, fulminant hepatic failure, Reye's syndrome, and metabolic encephalopathies.

Neuro-Specific Monitoring

Accurate neurological assessment is fundamental for the management of patients with intracranial pathology. This consists of repeated clinical examinations (particularly GCS and pupillary response) and the use of specific monitoring techniques, including serial CT scans of the brain. This chapter provides an overview of the more common monitoring modalities found within the neurocritical care environment.

In general terms, a combination of assessments is more likely to detect change than any one specific modality. Real-time continuous monitoring (e.g., measurement of intracranial pressure, ICP) will provide more timely warning about adverse events (e.g., an expanding hematoma) compared to static assessments such as sedation holds or serial CT brain scans.

Clinical Assessment

The Glasgow Coma Scale

The Glasgow Coma Scale (GCS) provides a standardized and internationally recognized method for evaluating a patient's CNS function by recording their best response to verbal and physical stimuli. A drop of two or more GCS points (or one or more motor points) should prompt urgent re-evaluation and a repeat CT scan.

Eye opening is not synonymous with awareness, and can be seen in both coma and persistent vegetative state (PVS). The important detail is that the patients either open their eyes to a specific command or shows ability to fix eye on a specific target or follows a visual stimulus.

Pupillary response

Changes in pupil size and reaction may provide useful additional information:
- Sudden unilateral fixed pupil: Compression of the third nerve, e.g., ipsilateral uncal herniation or posterior communicating artery aneurysm
- Unilateral miosis: Horner syndrome (consider vascular injury)
- Bilateral miosis: Narcotics, pontine hemorrhage
- Bilateral fixed, dilated pupils: Brainstem death, massive overdose (e.g., tricyclic antidepressants)

In the non-specialist center, neurological assessment of the ventilated patient consists of serial CT brain scans, pupillary response, and assessment of GCS during sedation holds. A reduction in sedation level will usually be at the suggestion of the Regional Neurosurgical Center (RNC) and its timing will depend upon a number of factors. Responses such as unilateral pupillary dilatation, extensor posturing, seizures, or severe hypertension should prompt rapid re-sedation, repeat CT scan, and contact with the RNC. In the patient with multiple injuries, consideration must be given to their analgesic requirements prior to any decrease in sedation levels.

Invasive Monitoring

Cerebral perfusion pressure (CPP) reflects the pressure gradient that drives cerebral blood flow (CBF), and hence cerebral oxygen delivery. Measurement of intracranial pressure (ICP) allows estimation of CPP. CPP is mean arterial pressure minus ICP.

Sufficient CPP is needed to allow CBF to meet the metabolic requirements of the brain. An inadequate CPP may result in the failure of autoregulation of flow to meet metabolic needs whilst an artificially induced high CPP may result in hyperemia and vasogenic edema, thereby worsening ICP. The CPP needs to be assessed for each individual and other monitoring modality (e.g., jugular venous oximetry, brain tissue oxygenation) may be required to assess its adequacy.

Despite its almost universal acceptance, there are no properly controlled trials demonstrating improved outcome from either ICP- or CPP-targeted therapy. However, in the early 1990s Marmarou et al. showed that patients with ICP values consistently greater than 20 mmHg suffered worse outcomes than matched controls, and poorer outcomes have been described in patients, whose CPP dropped below 60 mmHg (Marmarou 1991; Juul 2000; Young 2003). As such, ICP- and CPP- targeted therapy have become an accepted standard of care in head injury management.

The 2007 Brain Trauma Foundation Guidelines (Brain Trauma Foundation 2007) recommend treating ICP values above

20 mmHg and to target CPP in the range of 50-70 mmHg.

Patients with intact pressure autoregulation will tolerate higher CPP values. Aggressive attempts to maintain CPP >70 mmHg should be avoided because of the risk of ARDS.

Table 6.1 – ICP Values

Normal ICP <15 mmHg
Focal ischemia occurs at ICP >20 mmHg Global ischemia occurs at ICP >50 mmHg Usual treatment threshold is 20 mmHg

Measuring ICP

Intraventricular devices consist of a drain inserted into the lateral ventricle via a burr hole, and connected to a pressure transducer, manometer, or fiber optic catheter. Although associated with a higher incidence of infection and greater potential for brain injury during placement, this remains the gold standard. It has the added benefit of allowing CSF drainage. Historically, saline could be injected to assess brain compliance.

Extraventricular systems are placed in parenchymal tissue, the subarachnoid space, or in the epidural space via a burr hole.

These can be inserted at the bedside in the ICU. These systems are tipped with a transducer requiring calibration, and are subject to drift (particularly after long-term placement).

Examples of extraventricular systems are the Codman and Camino devices. These devices have a tendency to underestimate ICP.

In general, both types of device are left *in situ* for as short a time as possible to minimize the risk of introducing infection. Prophylactic antibiotics are not generally used.

Indications for ICP monitoring

In any case of head injury, if brain CT is positive for

pathology, and the patient fulfills the criteria for use of a ventilator,

monitoring for intracranial pressure (ICP) becomes mandatory. More specific indications are shown in Table 6.2.

Table 6.2 – Indications for intracranial pressure (ICP) monitoring

1) Traumatic brain injury, in particular:
   - Severe head injury (GCS<8)
   - Focal pathology on CT brainscan
   - Head injury and age >40
   - Normal CT brain scan but systolic blood pressure persistently <90 mmHg
   - Where other injuries and their treatment necessitate the use of sedation or anesthesia
2) Subarachnoid hemorrhage with associated hydrocephalus
3) Hydrocephalus
4) Hypoxic brain injury, for example, after near-drowning
5) Postoperative in patients at risk of severe cerebral edema
6) Encephalopathy (e.g., in liver failure)

Coagulopathy is the primary contraindication to insertion. The ICP device will generally be removed as soon as the patient is awake with satisfactory neurology (GCS motor score M5 or M6) or when physiological challenges (removal of sedation, normalizing $PaCO_2$) no longer produce a sustained rise in ICP.

Intracranial Pressure Waveforms and Analysis

The normal ICP waveform is a modified arterial trace and consists of three characteristic peaks. The "percussive" P_1 wave results from arterial pressure being transmitted from the choroid plexi, the "tidal" P_2 wave varies with brain compliance, whilst P_3 represents the dicrotic notch and closure of the aortic valve. It is important to establish the accuracy of the ICP trace and value before initiating therapy based upon the numbers generated. Transient sequential occlusion of the internal jugular veins or removing the head-up tilt should produce an increase in ICP.

The ICP waveform: The ICP waveform can be divided into systolic and diastolic components and demonstrates cardiac and respiratory variations.

- P1 (percussion wave): originates from pulsations in choroid plexus, sharp peak, consistent in amplitude
- P2 (tidal wave): variable in shape, ends on dicrotic notch
- P3 (dicrotic wave): begins immediately after dicrotic notch When ICP increases and compliance decreases, P_2 and P_3 elevate

causing a rounder waveform.

In addition to simple pressure measurement, if ICP is recorded against time, a number of characteristic wave forms (Lundeberg waves) can be seen.

- A waves: Pathological sustained plateau waves of 50-80 mmHg lasting between 5 and 10 min, possibly representing cerebral vasodilatation and an increase in CBF response to a low CPP.
- B waves: Small, transient waves of limited amplitude every 1-2 min representing fluctuations in cerebral blood volume. These may be seen in normal subjects, but are indicative of intracranial pathology when the amplitude increases above 10 mmHg.
- C waves: Small oscillations in ICP that reflect changes in systemic arterial pressure.

With cerebral autoregulation intact, a rise in MAP produces vasoconstriction and a fall in ICP. However, when autoregulation fails, the circulation becomes pressure passive and changes in MAP are reflected in changes in the ICP. Continuous analysis of MAP and ICP allows a correlation coefficient called the pressure reactivity index to be derived (PRx). Positive values indicate disturbed cerebral vascular reactivity, whilst negative values indicate that reactivity remains intact (Gupta 2002).

Despite the fact that trial results have not always been compelling, most clinicians regard the ICP monitor as an essential tool that allows estimation of CPP (Czosnyka 2004; Czosnyka 1996), gives early warning of developing pathology, allows the response to therapy to be objectively measured, and has value as a prognostic indicator (Joseph 2005).

Methods of intracranial pressure ICP measurement: Methods for the measurement of intracranial pressure are ventriculostomy, subdural catheter, epidural transducer, and fiberoptic microtransducer. Ventriculostomy remains the gold standard for monitoring ICP as it offers an accurate and reliable means of calibration. Disadvantages include a <2% risk for infection, a <10% risk for hemorrhage and difficulty in placing the catheter (Clark 1989).

One of the widely used forms of ICP monitoring is the fiberoptic or bolt ICP monitor. This method is relatively less invasive with lower morbidity. It lacks, however therapeutic CSF drainage.

Steps to ICP bolt placement (Crutchfeld 1990):

1. ICP bolt placement takes place in the ICU or the OR
2. A small skin incision to the skull bone is made
3. The periosteum is stripped off the bone and a drill burr hole is made to match the size of a bolt adapter. The bolt screw is then advanced into the skull and a dilator is used to dilate a tract in the dura for the fiberoptic probe
4. The skin is closed around the bolt
5. The fiberoptic probe is zeroed at atmospheric pressure
6. The probe is then placed through a retaining cap into

the subarachnoid space or less commonly intraparenchymally

7. Probe placement can be verified by observing ICP waveforms

8. The ICP monitor is then connected to the bedside monitorFiberoptic transducers cannot be recalibrated externally.

Table 6.3 – Comparison between fiberoptic ICP monitoring and ventriculostomy (Andrew 2010)

	Fiberoptic bolt	Ventriculostomy
Accuracy	Subject to shift	Gold standard
Placement	Relatively easy	Relatively hard
Feasibility of use	No recalibration	Requires height adjustment and zeroing
Clinical use	Measurement only	Measurement and CSF draining
ICP measurement	Focal pressure variation is a disadvantage	Focal variation disadvantage is less
Continuous care	Lower burden	Higher burden
Risk of infection	Lower	Increases after >5 days

ICP waveform analysis: Analysis of the relationship between ICP waveforms and ABP waveforms, i.e., pressure reactivity index (PRx), has been outlined (Czosnyka 1996).

1. PRx varies from low values (no correlation) to values approaching 1.0 (strong correlation)
2. With lower BP, lower blood vessel wall tension results in an increase in transmission of the BP waveform to the ICP
3. With elevated ICP brain compliance is reduced thus increasing the transmission of the BP waveform

Approximate Entropy (ApEn) is a logarithmic measure of system regularity or randomness that can be used in physiologic systems (Pincus 1991). Reductions in ApEn imply reduced randomness or increased order and may indicate pathology in the cardiovascular, respiratory and endocrine systems.

Cerebral blood flow CBF measurement is feasible and may be considered in some patients. On the other hand, cerebral tissue metabolic demand is not currently available.

Indirect measures of CBF include measurement of surrogates of cerebral tissue physiology as jugular venous oxygen saturation, tissue oxygen tension, and microdialysis. Other indirect markers for CBF measurement include cerebral perfusion pressure (CPP) and less directly continuous EEG.

Jugular Venous Oximetry ($SjvO_2$)

$SjvO_2$ is an indicator of global oxygen extraction of the brain. Jugular venous desaturation suggests an increase in cerebral oxygen extraction which indirectly implies that there has been a decrease in cerebral oxygen delivery, and hence perfusion.

The internal jugular vein drains the majority of blood from the brain, and in most patients the right lateral sinus is larger.

Despite the fact that flow is different on the two sides, oxygen saturations are normally very similar. This also appears to be the case in diffuse brain injury, whilst in focal injuries there tends to be a greater difference in the saturation of the two veins.

Jugular venous saturation can be measured using the principle of infrared refractometry via a specially designed catheter (Gopinath 1994). $SjvO_2$ values are:
- 55-75% - normal
- >75% - luxury perfusion
- <54% hypoperfusion
- <40% suggests global ischemia and is associated

with increased cerebral lactate production.

Insertion of Jugular Venous Saturation Catheter: Insertion involves retrograde cannulation of the internal jugular vein. A pediatric pulmonary artery catheter introducer can be used through which the fiber optic $SjvO_2$ catheter is advanced beyond the outlet of the common facial vein to the level of the jugular bulb at the base of the skull. Ultrasound is often used for accurate identification of vein position to avoid arterial puncture, and to minimize the risk of hematoma formation which can in turn impede venous drainage. Correct positioning is confirmed on a lateral neck X-ray with the catheter tip lying at the level of the mastoid air cells.

Indications for $SjvO_2$ Monitoring:

– Acute brain injury. An association between SjvO2 desaturation and poor neurological outcome has been observed. Fandino showed that in traumatic head injury SjvO2 was the only factor associated with outcome, whilst Gopinath showed that multiple SjvO2 desaturations were associated with an increased incidence of poor neurological outcome compared to those who showed no desaturations (Moppett 2004).

– Optimal CPP would appear to be at the point when further increases in MAP do not lead to a rise in SjvO2.

– Monitoring of therapy response. If ICP and SjvO2 are both raised, hyperemia is implied and hyperventilation is appropriate. SjvO2 should be monitored and kept above 55% in these circumstances, as excessive hyperventilation may cause profound cerebral vasoconstriction and cerebral ischemia. More recent work using PET scanning, however, has cast some doubt on the value of SjvO2, with hyperventilation appearing to increase ischemic brain volume without necessarily producing a fall in jugular venous saturation.

– To guide optimal blood pressure and PaCO2 management during operative treatment of aneurysms following SAH. During the operative treatment of an aneurysm, hypertension must be avoided because of the risk of rupture and bleeding. However, excessive reductions in blood pressure may risk cerebral ischemia, especially in those patients with preoperative hypertension. SjvO2 monitoring allows the anesthetist to assess the degree to which blood pressure can be safely lowered during the operative period. Similarly, a low PaCO2 will cause SjvO2 desaturation.

Problems with SjvO$_2$ Monitoring: The major criticism of SjvO$_2$ is that it is a measure of global oxygen delivery and does not reflect metabolic inadequacies in focal areas of injury and hence may miss regional areas of ischemia. Inaccuracies can occur with catheter misplacement, contamination with extra cerebral blood, when the catheter abuts the vessel wall, or if thrombosis occurs around the catheter tip. Contraindications and complications are similar to those of an IJV central line.

Interpretation of Changes in SjvO$_2$:

If cerebral oxygen delivery is impaired, oxygen extraction increases and SjvO$_2$ decreases. If autoregulation is intact, CBF increases to meet metabolic demand and SjvO$_2$ is restored.

However, in the injured brain autoregulation is often impaired and cerebral ischemia ensues.

- Decreased SjvO2: This implies inadequate cerebral oxygen delivery that may be due to decreased oxygen delivery (systemic hypoxia, anemia), decreased CBF (hypotension, raised ICP, excessive hypocapnia or vasospasm), or increased cerebral oxygen consumption (seizures, hyperthermia, pain)
- Increased SjvO2: This is somewhat more difficult to interpret, and may represent either hyperemia (e.g., when the autoregulation mechanisms are lost) or reduced oxygen consumption (e.g., hypothermia, deep

sedation, or cerebral infarction).
- Lactate Oxygen Index: During cerebral hypoperfusion the brain can become a net producer of lactate, with the jugular venous lactate rising above arterial values.

Brain Tissue Oximetry

Interest in measuring brain tissue oxygenation via implantable sensors has grown in recent years. The Licox sensor is an implantable polarographic electrode that measures tissue oxygen tensions. It is inserted through a compatible bolt and ideally should be placed into the penumbral area of the injury. Oxygen diffuses from the tissue through the catheter into an electrolyte chamber where an electrical current is generated. Brain tissue oxygen tension is normally lower than arterial oxygen tension (15-50 mmHg); whilst tissue CO_2 is normally higher (range 40-70 mmHg). The sensors are useful in monitoring local changes and trends in tissue oxygenation that might be missed by $SjvO_2$ measurements.

At present it is primarily used in severe head injury and poor-grade subarachnoid hemorrhage, and in conjunction with other monitoring modalities. The technique allows a continuous method of monitoring of regional tissue oxygenation and in particular, monitoring areas of high ischemic risk, and is a promising and reliable clinical tool.

Direct measures of CBF:

Measurement of injectable tracers that reach the brain after peripheral injection using signal intensity changes.

Xenon-Enhanced CT:

In this technique xenon, a diffusible agent is used. The patient inhales a mixture of 28% xenon and 72% oxygen for approximately 4 minutes after baseline CT scans are obtained. Sequential scanning of the same slices occurs during the inhalation period. Tissue attenuation vs. time data is then obtained. The arterial concentration is proportional to the expired xenon concentration. Advantages are the relatively low cost and high ease of use. The downside is a high sensitivity to motion artifact (Andrew 2010).

SPECT (Single Photo Emission CT):

In SPECT scanning, the radioisotope technetium-99m (Tc-99m) is combined with hexamethylpropyleneamine (HMPAO) or ethyl cysteinate dimer.

SPECT scanning has the advantage of being easy to perform. However, there are limitations with regards to assembly of the compound.

MR Perfusion: "Dynamic Susceptibility Contrast Imaging" also called "first-pass" or "bolus tracking" MR perfusion imaging is based on rapid acquisition of MR signal intensity data from the brain during the injection of a contrast agent. Signal intensity-

time curves are generated for each pixel in the image then CBF is calculated.

Noninvasive Monitoring

Continuous measures of CBF by Transcranial Doppler

Transcranial Doppler (TCD) is a noninvasive technique that calculates blood flow velocity in the cerebral vasculature. An ultrasound beam is reflected back by the moving bloodstream at a different frequency than it was transmitted (Doppler shift), and from the Doppler equation, the velocity of blood flow (FV) can be calculated. Changes in FV correlate well with changes in CBF, as long as the orientation of the transducer and the vessel diameter remain constant. It is used clinically to diagnose vasospasm, to test cerebral autoregulation, and to detect emboli during cardiac surgery and carotid endarterectomy (Moppett 2004).

Normal Values. From the FV waveform systolic, diastolic, and mean velocities can be calculated. The mean FV in the middle cerebral artery (MCA) is usually 35-90 cm/s and correlates well with CBF. The FV can be influenced by age, being lowest at birth (24 cm/s), highest at age 4-6 years (100 cm/s), and then declining until the seventh decade of life (40 cm/s). FV is also 3-5% higher in females and increases in hemodilutional states.

Technique for Insonating the Middle Cerebral Artery (MCA): The M1 branch of the MCA is the commonest vessel to be insonated, and is visualized through a transtemporal window with a 2 MHz pulsed Doppler signal. The anterior and posterior cerebral arteries can also be accessed through this window, whilst a transorbital approach allows access to the carotid siphon and the suboccipital route to the basilar and vertebral arteries.

Analysis of Doppler waveform: Analysis of the Doppler waveform gives rise to useful derived variables as well as blood velocity information.
- Pulsatility Index (PI): $FV_{sys}-FV_{dias}/FV_{mean}$ (normal value: 0.6-1.1). This reflects distal cerebrovascular resistance and correlates with CPP.
- Change in CBF with arterial CO_2 tension (cerebral vascular reactivity).

Uses of TCD in Intensive Care Head Injury: Three distinct phases have been shown in severe head injury with regard to CBF and MCA FV.
- Phase 1 occurs on the day of injury and has a normal CBF, normal MCA FV, and normal AVDO2.
- Phase 2 occurring 1-2 days post-injury, a hyperemic state is encountered with an increased CBF, MCA FV and decreased AVDO2.
- The final phase seen at days 4-15 is the vasospastic phase and is associated with a significantly decreased CBF and increased MCA FV. The use of TCD allows interpretation of the dynamic physiological changes

seen in severe head injury, and in combination with other modalities allows perfusion and oxygenation to be optimized for the individual patient.

The highest MCA FV recorded at any stage is an independent predictor of outcome from head injury, and the loss of autoregulation (calculated by regression of CPP on MCA FV) has also been shown to be a predictor of poor outcome from head injury.

Subarachnoid Hemorrhage: Vasospasm occurs in approximately 50% of people with subarachnoid hemorrhage between 2-17 days post-event, and is associated with significant morbidity and mortality. TCD may be used to detect vasospasm by the increase in MCA FV associated with vessel narrowing.

Spasm is also assumed to be occurring when blood velocity is >120 cm/s. High MCA FV is associated with worse-grade SAH, larger blood loads on CT (assessed by Fisher Grade) and hence worse outcome (Steiger 1994).

Near Infrared Spectroscopy

While the criticism of jugular venous oximetry is that it is representative of global oxygen delivery, near infrared spectroscopy (NIRS) is a noninvasive technique that measures regional cerebral oxygenation.

Light in the near infrared wavelength (700-1,000 nm) can pass through bone, skin, and other tissues with minimal absorption, but is partly scattered and partly absorbed by brain tissue. The amount of light absorbed is proportional to the concentration of chromophobes (iron in hemoglobin, and copper in cytochromes), and measurement of absorption at a number of wavelengths provides an estimate of oxygenation (Owen-Reece 1999).

The probes illuminate a volume of about 8-10 ml of tissue and are ideally suited for use in neonates because of their thin skull, but have been used with success in adults.

Advantages of this technique are that it is non-invasive, and provides a regional indicator of cerebral oxygenation. Its major limitation is its inability to distinguish between intra- and extra- cranial changes in blood flow.

Electrophysiological Monitoring

An electroencephalogram (EEG) is obtained using the standardized system of electrode placement. Practically, this is not often readily available and requires expert interpretation. The EEG is affected by anesthetic agents and physiological abnormalities such as hypoxia, hypoperfusion and hypercarbia.

A number of methods have been developed to simplify and summarize the EEG data:
- Cerebral Function Monitor (CFM): This is a modified device from a conventional EEG. It uses a single biparietal or bitemporal lead, and is processed to give an overall representation of average cortical activity.
- Cerebral function analyzing monitor: Developed from the CFM but displays information about amplitude and frequency separately.
- Bispectral Analysis: This modification of the EEG analyzes the phase and power between any two EEG frequencies. The bispectral index (BIS) is a dimensionless number statistically derived from these phased and power frequencies and ranges from 0 to 100 (100-awake, 60-unconscious, 0- isoelectric EEG). This technology was derived with normal subjects and is not readily transferable to the injured brain, but may have a use in guiding sedation and analgesia.

Spectral Edge Frequency: Compressed Spectral Array: Raw EEG data is processed into a number of sine waves (Fourier analysis). Power spectral analysis then investigates the relationship between power and frequency of the sine waves over a short time period (Epoch). The compressed spectral array is obtained by superimposing linear plots of successive epochs to produce a three-dimensional "hill and valley" plot. The spectral edge frequency looks at the frequency below which a determined power of the total power spectrum occurs. SEF90 indicates a spectral edge frequency of 90% and is the frequency below which 90% of activity is occurring.

Continuous Electroencephalogram Monitoring: When a comatose, critically ill patient arrives in the intensive care unit (ICU), he is connected to a pulse oximetry monitor, ECG monitor, respiration monitor, arterial blood pressure monitor, etc, to provide physicians and nurses with real-time information about cardiopulmonary physiology. Monitoring for the brain has been unavailable to ICU staff until recently.

In comatose or sedated patients, there may be too few examination findings that can be reliably followed to assess worsening brain injury. Neuroimaging cannot reveal functional changes, such as seizures and level of sedation; it provides information about structural brain injury often after it is irreversible. There is great need for central nervous system monitoring for at-risk patients, as more interventions are becoming available to manage neurologic injury and "time is brain".

It is now possible to monitor and record the continuous digital electroencephalogram, with full electrode placement, of many critically ill patients simultaneously. Continuous EEG monitoring (cEEG) provides real-time dynamic information about brain function, which is especially useful when the clinical examination is limited. Nonconvulsive seizures and nonconvulsive status epilepticus are common in comatose critically ill patients and can have multiple negative effects on the injured brain.

Nonconvulsive status epilepticus (NCSE) seems to be an important issue in stroke; NCSE is a frequent finding reaching 18% in a recent multicenter study (Kitchener 2010), thus requiring a high degree of suspicion in an acute stroke setting to avoid further neuronal injury and morbidity. The majority of seizure activity in these patients cannot be detected without cEEG. So, cEEG monitoring is mandatory to detect and guide management of nonconvulsive status, including those that occur following convulsive status epilepticus. In addition, it is used to guide management of pharmacological coma sometimes used for treatment of increased intracranial pressure. There are emerging applications for cEEG, one of which is to detect new or worsening brain ischemia in patients at high risk, especially those with subarachnoid hemorrhage. As qEEG software is continuously improving, full scalp cEEG monitoring is feasible, and can provide continuous information about changes in brain function in real time at the bedside and to alert clinicians to any acute brain event, including seizures, ischemia, increasing intracranial pressure, hemorrhage, and even systemic abnormalities affecting the brain, such as hypoxia, hypotension, acidosis, and others. cEEG monitoring without expert review of the raw EEG, must not be allowed as false positives and false negatives are common. When cEEG is combined with individualized multimodality brain monitoring, intensivists can identify when the brain is at risk for injury or when neuronal injury is already occurring and intervene before there is permanent damage. We believe that cEEG has significant potential to improve neurologic outcomes in a variety of settings.

Application of the EEG in the ICU:
- Seizure management: Confirms the diagnosis of seizures and identifies a focal or lateralized source of activity. It also helps to distinguish between involuntary movements, posturing, and eye signs that are common in intensive care and true seizure activity.

- Nonconvulsive status epilepticus (NCSE): This represents a state that lasts more than 30 min with clinical evidence in alteration in mental state from normal, and seizure activity on the EEG. Between 4 and 20% of patients with status epilepticus have nonconvulsive episodes. NCSE is a frequent finding in ischemic stroke reaching 18% of ischemic stroke patients admitted to neurocritical care units.
- Metabolic suppression: Burst suppression (isoelectric EEG) is a definable end point when pharmacological reduction of the cerebral metabolic rate of the injured brain is required for either neuroprotection or intractable intracranial hypertension.
- Ensuring adequate sedation in patients who require prolonged neuromuscular paralysis.
- Prognosis: The EEG can be of prognostic value following brain injury, with absence of spontaneous variability being associated with poor outcome.

Multimodal Monitoring

In any type of brain injury, the available monitoring modalities are prone to artifact and misinterpretation. By utilizing more than one monitoring technique, the observer is more likely to determine whether a genuine change in cerebral physiology has occurred and what the most appropriate intervention should be. For instance, in traumatic brain-injured patients we routinely monitor ICP, processed EEG, $SjvO_2$ and brain-tissue oxygen tension ($PbtO_2$), allowing us to observe both local and regional changes in cerebral hemodynamics. General rules cannot always be applied to individual patients, and multimodal monitoring can allow more informed decision making such as determining CPP thresholds or the ability of the cerebral vasculature to autoregulate (Cecil 2011; Czosnyka 1996).

Conclusions

A wide range of monitoring techniques is available, each with different strengths and limitations. Multimodal monitoring using a combination of techniques can overcome some of the limitations of the individual methods discussed. The choice of monitoring is often guided by clinical familiarity and local policy.

Key points:
1. Repeated clinical assessment through the Glasgow Coma Scale (GCS) is the cornerstone of neurological evaluation.
2. Ventilated head-injured patients with intracranial pathology on CT require ICP monitoring.
3. Invasive or non-invasive neurospecific monitoring requires careful interpretation when assisting goal-directed therapies.
4. Multimodal monitoring using a combination of techniques can overcome some of the limitations of individual methods.

7. Cerebral Edema
NAbil Kitchener

Cerebral edema is a challenging problem in the neurocritical care setting. Different etiologies may cause increased intracranial pressure. Secondary brain injury may ensue as a result of cerebral edema, and may result in different herniation syndromes.

Brain monitoring for increased intracranial pressure may by employed in certain patient populations. Serial neuroimaging may be useful in monitoring exacerbations of brain edema.

Osmotherapy has been recommended for management of cerebral edema. Mannitol and hypertonic saline are the two agents widely used for this purpose. Knowledge of possible side effects of osmotherapeutic agents is necessary. Common concerns of such therapies include renal insufficiency, pulmonary edema, and exacerbation of congestive heart failure, hypernatremia, hemolysis, and hypotension. Specific measures as controlled ventilation, sedation and analgesia, pharmacologic coma, hypothermia and surgical decompression may be required in patient subpopulations. Important questions still need to be answered regarding the timing of the decompressive surgery and patient selection criteria.

Surgical decompression may be applicable in certain patients. Recent studies indicate that surgical decompression may significantly reduce mortality in young patients with malignant cerebral infarcts.

General medical management is focused toward limiting secondary brain damage. General measures include head and neck position, optimization of cerebral perfusion and oxygenation, management of fever, nutritional support and glycemic control.

Abnormalities of intracranial pressure may result in pathology requiring urgent evaluation and intervention to prevent life- threatening consequences. This pathology may represent intracranial hyper- or hypotension, or it may manifest as an abnormality of cerebrospinal fluid (CSF) dynamics, such as hydrocephalus. Elevated intracerebral pressure is the final common pathway for almost all pathology leading to brain death, and interventions to treat ICP may preserve life and improve neurologic function after head trauma, stroke, or other neurologic emergencies.

Common causes of raised intracranial pressure are shown in Table 7.1, symptoms and signs in Table 7.2.

Table 7.1 – Some common causes of increased intracranial pressure (Czosnyka 1999)

Head injury	Intracranial hematoma (extradural, subdural, and intracerebral)
	Diffuse brain swelling
	Contusion
Cerebrovascular	Subarachnoid hemorrhage
	Intracerebral hematoma
	Cerebral venous thrombosis Major cerebral infarct
	Hypertensive encephalopathy (malignant hypertension, eclampsia)
Hydrocephalus	Congenital or acquired
	Obstructive or communicating
Craniocerebral disproportion	Brain "tumour" (cysts; benign or malignant tumours)
	Secondary hydrocephalus
	Mass effect
	Oedema
	"Benign" intracranial hypertension (pseudotumor cerebri; idiopathic intracranial hypertension)
CNS infection	Meningitis
	Encephalitis
	Abscess
	Cerebral malaria
Metabolic encephalopathy	Hypoxic-ischemic
	Reye's syndrome, etc.
	Lead encephalopathy
	Hepatic coma
	Renal failure
	Diabetic ketoacidosis Burns
	Near drowning
	Hyponatremia
	Status epilepticus

Types of Cerebral Edema

Cerebral swelling or edema can complicate many intracranial pathologic processes including neoplasms, hemorrhage, trauma, autoimmune diseases, hyperemia, or ischemia. There are essentially three types of cerebral

edema:
1. Cytotoxic edema is associated with cell death and failure of ion homeostasis. Cytotoxic edema results from energy failure of a cell as a result of hypoxic or ischemic stress,

    which leads to cell death. Intracellular swelling occurs and results in the CT and MR appearance of both gray and white matter edema, usually in the distribution of a vascular or borderzone territory after hypoxia or stroke.
2. Vasogenic edema is associated with breakdown of the blood-brain barrier. Vasogenic edema represents breakdown of the blood-brain barrier, appears mostly in the white matter, and is more likely to be associated with neoplasms or cerebral abscesses. In reality, cerebral edema in many situations, usually exhibit a combination of vasogenic and cytotoxic edema.
3. Interstitial (hydrostatic or hydrocephalic) edema is associated with hydrocephalus, in which there is increased tension of CSF across the ependyma. Interstitial edema, or transependymal flow, is radiographically seen with hypodense areas surrounding the ventricular system and is associated with increased CSF volume or pressure.

Table 7.2 – Signs and symptoms of increased intracranial pressure and edema

Symptoms	Physical Signs

Headache, worsened with Valsalva	Progressive decline in level of consciousness
Decreased visual acuity	Decreased upward gaze
Diplopia	Cranial nerve VI palsy
Nausea	Papilledema
Vomiting	Loss of normal venous pulsations in the fundus
	Field cut or enlarged physiologic blind spot
	Alterations in vital signs

Management of Cerebral Edema

The treatment of cerebral edema depends mainly on treating the underlying cause. In cytotoxic edema, osmotic therapy with mannitol and hypertonic saline may not reduce edema in the lesion itself, but may reduce the volume of normal brain allowing for some increased margin of safety by decreasing intracranial pressure (Raslan 2007). Steroids are of no value in cytotoxic edema due to stroke, and may be harmful in the settings of brain trauma. Surgical decompression of cytotoxic edema with decompressive craniectomy may be therapeutic, and life-saving (Hofmeijer 2009). Vasogenic edema responds to steroids and surgical resection of the lesion, and may also benefit from osmotic therapy with mannitol or hypertonic saline (Oddo 2009). Hydrostatic edema is treated surgically with CSF removal or shunting, and it is treated medically with agents to decrease production of CSF, such as acetazolamide and furosemide.

8. General Neurological Treatment Strategies

MAGdy KhALAf, NABil Kitchener

The concept of neurocritical care has been developed to coordinate the management of critically ill neurological patients within a single specialist unit and to include clinical situations such as swallowing disturbances, respiratory problems management in neurocritical care, infection control in the unit, pain relief and sedation in some patients, as well as diagnosing brain death. Acute rehabilitation is important in securing improved long-term neurological outcomes after many brain insults, trauma, ischemia or hemorrhage. Intervention from neurophysiotherapists, as part of the neurocritical care multiprofessional team, must occur as early as possible.

Respiratory muscle impairment is the most common reason for admission to the ICU in patients with neuromuscular disorders. Objective measures of respiratory muscle function are necessary because significant respiratory muscle impairment may exist despite a paucity of symptoms.

Analgesia in the neurocritical care unit is indicated in many situations such as postoperative pain, traumatic injury, and subacute or chronic pains. Although it is mandatory and beneficial in many situations, precautions must be taken before

applying many agents; e.g., equipment and personnel to intubate and mechanically ventilate patients must be readily available with use of narcotic agonists. Some agents may cause decreased level of consciousness or obtundation leading to impairment of neurological exam. This chapter will cover management of these issues in the neurocritical care setting.

Swallowing Disturbances

Weakness, spasticity or both of the pharynx and tongue cause dysphagia and tendency for aspiration. A feeding tube through a percutaneous endoscopic gastrostomy (PEG), cervical esophagostomy or jejunostomy is a reliable method of patient feeding when prolonged deficit is expected. Nutrition support by enteral feeding through either a nasogastric or an orogastric tube should be maintained in all intubated patients whenever possible. In patients with a normal baseline nutritional state, support should be initiated within 7 days. In malnourished patients, nutritional support should be initiated within 72 h.

Delayed gastric emptying is common in critically ill patients on sedative medications but often responds to promotility agents such as domperidone, and metoclopramide (Gomes 2010).

Parenteral nutrition is an alternative to enteral nutrition in patients with severe gastrointestinal pathology. When patients improve the gastrostomy is easy to close. It is better to try to provide adequate and safe nutrition by mouth in an alert patient before placing a feeding tube. Nasogastric tubes have been used temporarily for feeding but they are uncomfortable, cause pressure necrosis of the nares when used chronically, and allow aspiration, so it should not be used for long. In ambulatory patients with severe dysphagia, cervical esophagostomy may be useful, as a patient can insert the tube during feedings and the ostium can be covered with a dressing at other times. Patients with severe weakness or ataxia of the upper extremities are usually unable to feed themselves, so percutaneous endoscopic gastrostomy is the method of choice (Wanklyn 1995). Tube

feeding needs high caloric diet (1200 to 2400 Kcal/day) for active patients, and liquid foods are usually concentrated to deliver
1 Kcal/ml. To avoid clogging of the tube, each feeding is followed with water. Tube feeding is best started with about one half the total desired calories diluted in water, with gradual increase in concentration and calories, to avoid diarrhea and malabsorption, reaching a maximum volume of about 200 ml (150 ml food and 50 ml of water). If aspiration of saliva and nasal secretions is a problem, a cuffed endotracheal tube is necessary and the use of tricyclic antidepressants or anticholinergic drugs (if there is no absolute contraindication for its use) might reduce salivation and prevent drooling (Fjærtoft 2011). Adequate nutritional feeding, trace elements, minerals and vitamins constitute the most important basic brain supplements.

Respiratory Management in Neurocritical Care

Most patients who are started on ventilatory support receive synchronized intermittent mandatory ventilation (SIMV), because this ensures user-specified backup minute ventilation in the event that the patient fails to initiate respiratory efforts.

Once the intubated patient has been stabilized with respect to oxygenation, definitive therapy for the underlying process responsible for respiratory failure is formulated and initiated. Subsequent modifications in ventilator therapy must be provided in parallel with changes in the patient's clinical status. As improvement in respiratory function is noted, the first priorities are to reduce PEEP and supplemental O_2 and once a patient can achieve adequate arterial saturation with an FIO_2

≤0.5 and 5 cm H_2O PEEP, attempts should be made to reduce the level of mechanical ventilatory support and weaning should be planned and started. Patients previously on full ventilator support should be switched to a ventilator mode that allows for weaning, such as SIMV, PSV (pressure support ventilation), or SIMV combined with PSV. Ventilator therapy can then be gradually removed while patients whose condition continues to

deteriorate after ventilator support is initiated may require increased O_2, PEEP, and alternative modes of ventilation such as IRV or OLV (Borel 2000). Patients who are started on mechanical ventilation usually require some form of sedation and analgesia to maintain an acceptable level of comfort. Often, this regimen consists of a combination of a benzodiazepine and opiate administered intravenously. Medications commonly used for this purpose include lorazepam, midazolam, diazepam, morphine, and fentanyl. Immobilized patients in the intensive care unit on mechanical ventilatory support are at increased risk for deep venous thrombosis; accepted practice consists of administering prophylaxis in the form of subcutaneous heparin and/or pneumatic compression boots. Fractionated low-molecular-weight heparin has also been used for this purpose; it appears to be equally effective and is associated with a decreased incidence of heparin-associated thrombocytopenia (Pelosi 2011).

Prophylaxis against diffuse gastrointestinal mucosal injury is indicated for patients who have suffered a neurologic insult, so histamine receptor antagonists (H_2 receptor antagonists), proton pump inhibitors, and cytoprotective agents such as Carafate have all been used for this purpose and appear to be effective.

Recent data suggest that Carafate use is associated with a reduction in the incidence of nosocomial pneumonias, since it does not cause changes in stomach PH and is less likely to permit colonization of the gastrointestinal tract by nosocomial organisms at neutral PH.

Endotracheal intubation and positive-pressure mechanical ventilation have direct and indirect effects on several organ systems, including the lung and upper airways, the cardiovascular system, and the gastrointestinal system. Pulmonary complications include barotraumas, nosocomial pneumonia, oxygen toxicity, tracheal stenosis, and deconditioning of respiratory muscles (Hurford 2002).

Upper airway function must be intact for a patient to remain extubated but is difficult to assess in the intubated patient.

Therefore, if a patient can breathe on his own, through an endotracheal tube, but develops stridor or recurrent aspiration once the tube is removed, upper airway dysfunction or an abnormal swallowing mechanism should be suspected, and plans for achieving a stable airway be developed. An intact cough reflex during suctioning is a good indicator of a patient's ability to mobilize secretions. Respiratory drive and chest wall functions are assessed by observation of respiratory rate, tidal volume, inspiratory pressure, and vital capacity (Hardin 2006). The weaning index, defined as the ratio of breathing frequency to tidal volume (breaths per minute per liter), is both sensitive and specific for predicting the likelihood of successful extubation. When this ratio is less than 105, and the patient can breathe without mechanical assistance through an endotracheal tube, successful extubation is likely. An inspiratory pressure of more than -30 cm H_2O and a vital capacity of greater than 10 ml/kg are considered indicators of acceptable chest wall and diaphragm functions. Alveolar ventilation is generally adequate when elimination of CO_2 is sufficient to maintain arterial pH in the range of 7.35 to 7.40, and SaO_2 >90% can be achieved with an FIO_2 <0.5 and a PEEP ≤5 cm H_2O. Although many patients may not meet all criteria for weaning, the likelihood that a patient will tolerate extubation without difficulty increases as more criteria are met (Hurford 2002).

Many approaches to wean patients from ventilator support have been advocated. T-piece and CPAP weaning are best tolerated by patients who have undergone mechanical ventilation for brief periods and require little respiratory muscle reconditioning, whereas SIMV and PSV are best for patients who have been intubated for extended periods and require gradual respiratory muscle reconditioning. Weaning by means of SIMV involves gradual tapering of the mandatory backup rate, in increments of 2 to 4 breaths per minute, while monitoring blood gas parameters and respiratory rates (Webb 1999). Rates of greater than 25 breaths per minute, on withdrawal of mandatory ventilator breaths, generally indicate respiratory muscle fatigue and the need to combine periods of exercise with periods of rest.

Exercise periods are gradually increased until a patient remains stable on SIMV at 4 breaths per minute or less without needing rest at higher SIMV rates. A CPAP or T-piece trial can then be attempted before planned extubation (Bernard 1994).

Infection Control in Neurocritical Care

Sepsis (and the systemic inflammatory response to sepsis) remains the major cause of organ failure and death in the intensive care unit, being either directly or indirectly responsible for 75% of all deaths (Valles 1997). Common sites of infection include the urinary tract, respiratory tract (especially ventilator associated pneumonia), vascular cannulae (catheter related sepsis) and long-term use of nasogastric feeding tubes. Vascular cannulae sepsis, particularly those associated with internal jugular and subclavian catheters, constitute the majority, but peripheral catheters also carry a considerable risk of infections. Thus, placement of intravenous lines requires careful aseptic technique and regular changing of lines. It is important to culture specimens from the tips of catheters that have been removed. Catheter related infections are usually caused by *StAphylococcus epidermidis* or *StAphylococcus Aureus*, and its treatment is empiric depending on use of vancomycin and cephalosporins.

Most nosocomial infections seen in the NICU are endogenous, caused by colonization of the patient's GI tract by pathogenic bacteria which then translocate through the intestinal mucosa to reach distant sites by hematogenous spread. With vascular cannulation, Gram-negative organisms such as *EscherichiA coli*, *KlebsieLLA*, and *PseudomonAS* species stated to be traditionally responsible, but Gram-positive organisms (*Streptococcus* and *StAphylococcus* species) are increasingly suspected. Fungi may also be implicated and considered the most serious infection (Vincent 1995).

Patients intubated for longer than 72 hours are at high risk for ventilator-associated pneumonia as a result of aspiration from the upper airways through small leaks around the endotracheal tube cuff; the most common organisms responsible for these conditions are enteric gram-negative rods, *StAphylococcus Aureus*, and anaerobic bacteria. Because the endotracheal tube and upper airways of patients on mechanical ventilation are commonly colonized with bacteria, the diagnosis of nosocomial pneumonia requires "protected brush" bronchoscopic sampling of airway secretions coupled with quantitative microbiologic techniques to differentiate colonization from infection.

Precautions and ways to combat nosocomial infections involve the isolation of the infected patient whenever possible, meticulous staff hygiene (hand washing before and after each patient contact, aseptic techniques for invasive procedures, etc), early identification and treatment of infection by the routine sending of blood, urine, sputum, etc, for culture, use of disposable equipments and, most importantly, joint daily ward rounds between microbiologists and the ICU team (Fagon 1993). Treatment of nosocomial infection, with or without septicemia, requires the administration of appropriate antibacterial drugs in adequate doses for an appropriate period.

Pain Relief and Sedation

In neurocritical care units different scores are used to evaluate patient anxiety, agitation and response to surroundings.

Different scores for pain, anxiety and agitation are used as guidelines for medication when pain is common, with a variety of causes such as anxiety, confusion, sleep deprivation, sepsis, drug withdrawal – especially sedatives, metabolic (hypo- or hyperglycemia, hypernatremia, uremia, hepatic precoma or coma), respiratory (infection, hypoxemia, hypercapnia) and cardiac (low output state, hypotension). It may manifest as discomfort, pulling at intravenous and bladder catheters, tracheal and nasogastric tubes, shouting, aggressive behavior, extreme restlessness, and confusion (Schnakers 2007). Pain is particularly common and often unrecognized because of confusion and the difficulties with communication in the aphonic, aphasic or paralyzed patient. Clinical assessment may direct attention through finding of profuse sweating, sustained tachycardia and blood pressure fluctuations, and dilated pupils. Most patients will require sedation but there is a natural reluctance to sedate patients with an evolving CNS disorder (McMillian 2011).

The first line of management is to reassure and calm the patient, ensuring a quiet environment and normal diurnal cycle. Next, there should be careful nursing and treatment of the underlying causes, including positioning, splinting, bed cages, catheterization, and physical treatments. In spite of reluctance to sedate patients with an evolving CNS disorder, sedative medications are mandatory and must be used, when indicated, to reduce pain, distress, and anxiety. Also they may be used to help patient toleration of tracheal tubes, IPPV, tracheal suction, and physiotherapy. Patients with neurologically-induced respiratory failure often require prolonged periods of mechanical ventilation in the NICU, and it is not desirable to keep such patients continuously sedated throughout their stay (Jacobi 2002). Furthermore, assessment of their condition and subsequent weaning is impossible when sedated. However, during periods of cardiorespiratory instability, raised ICP, and in cases of intubation, sedation may be essential. In the ICU environment, however, medications are often needed to calm patients. As many as 30 different medications are used, and the agents most frequently used are midazolam, olanzapine, propofol, lorazepam and opioid analgesics (Jacobi 2002).

Bedside approach to the agitated patient

Assess and manage immediate threat to life (airway, breathing, circulation and temperature).

Assess pain by querying the patient about pain, and assess for noxious stimuli after measurement of pain score. Correct any identified causes, and if the patient is hemodynamically unstable, give fentanyl 25-100 μgm IV q5-15 minutes until desired effect is achieved, or hydromorphone 0.25-0.75 mg IV q 5-15 minutes; if patient is hemodynamically stable, give morphine 2-5 mg IV every 5-15 minutes.

Assess anxiety. When patients have been on sedative and analgesic drug infusions for longer than 24 hours and begin to recover, daily interruptions of drug infusions for a time period sufficient to allow awakening is recommended (Blanchard 2002).

Role of Rehabilitation

Rehabilitation is a reiterative active, educational, problem- solving process, focused on the patient disability. The operational characteristics of rehabilitation services comprise a multidisciplinary group of people who work together towards common goals for each patient, involve and educate the patient and family in the process, have relevant expertise and experience (knowledge and skills) and can, between them, resolve most of the common problems faced by patients (Arnow 1993). The stages of rehabilitation involve general assessment to identify the nature and extent of the patient problems and the factors relevant to their solution, goal setting, then intervention, which may include treatments that affect the process of change and support (care), which maintain life and safety, and finally evaluation to check on the effects of the intervention.

The aims of rehabilitation are to maximize the participation of the patient in his/her social setting, minimize the pain and distress experienced by the patient and family and/or carers (Collen 1990). The development of models for disability has fostered and clarified discussion about the nature of rehabilitation. Definition of rehabilitation refers to the operational characteristics of a rehabilitation service (structure), how rehabilitation service works (process) and the aims of rehabilitation services (outcome).

Three specific core skills are particularly associated with rehabilitation:

1. An ability to assess all relevant aspects of patients' situation not simply their disease and its symptoms and signs, formulating the important interactions.

2. An ability to set realistic but challenging goals in both the short and long term, a skill that depends upon an accurate evaluation of the likely prognosis and scope for effective intervention.

3. An ability to participate in teamwork, working co-operatively with a group of other experts towards agreed common goals (Cunningham 2000).

However, recent research, mostly related to stroke, does support various hypotheses. First, there is now evidence that even quite small levels of intervention can have powerful and specific effects. There is also some evidence of a dose response relationship between therapeutic input and outcome. Second, there is some evidence that even the simple provision of information may be effective and acting on the patient's personal context is an important component of rehabilitation (Badley 1993). Third, patients should be encouraged to seek review of medication at regular intervals, perhaps every 6 months, especially for drugs that have cognitive side effects and either slow or hinder the process of recovery. Use drugs to treat specific impairments like gabapentin to improve visual acuity when nystagmus is present, and a dopamine agonist (such as bromocriptine) to ameliorate the reduced initiation after frontal lobe damage. Acute-onset disability is often considered the easiest to manage, because recovery occurs and may be complete (Wade 2000).

Diagnostic Findings in Cerebral Death

Brain death is the irreversible cessation of cerebral functions. Cerebral death, which is of medico-legal importance, cannot be accurately assessed on the basis of a criterion related to a single functional system. It is basically characterized by the absence of three main brain functions:

(1) Cerebral activity known as "cerebral responsivity"
(2) Vital functions
(3) Cephalic reflexes

Cephalic reflexes are mediated by the cranial nerves, and are considered as important indicators of the integrity of the brainstem, as absence of the cephalic reflexes are essential for considering the diagnosis of brain death, yet they differ in importance as a criterion of death. Some cephalic reflexes are considered to be the most sensitive and discriminative of brainstem functions, and accepted as criteria of cerebral brain death, e.g., pupillary reflex was absent in 98.4% of cases, corneal reflex was absent in practically all cases, and returns early if the patient shows any signs of survival (unless the cornea has become insensitive due to edema or dehydration), the oculocephalic reflex (Doll's eyes response) is quite discriminative, and it returns early, with evidence of recovery. The vestibular reflex is also quite discriminative for cerebral death, but upon recovery, it is slightly slower to return than the pupillary and corneal reflexes. The audio-ocular reflex, which is a blink of the eyelids in response to a sudden clap, is not as discriminative as the other cephalic reflexes, and is somewhat slower to recover. Snout reflex, pharyngeal (gag) reflex, swallowing reflex and cough reflex are not particularly discriminative.

In the collaborative study of cerebral death, absence of all cephalic reflexes was noted in more than half of the cases, whereas audio-ocular reflex was absent in 99% of cases, the pupillary reflex was absent in only 76.6%, and the audio-ocular reflex was extremely sensitive to brain injury.

Certain combinations of cranial nerve reflexes have been specified as essential for the diagnosis of brain death. The absence of pupillary, corneal, vestibular, audio-ocular and oculocephalic reflexes showed significant correlation with cerebral death (Smith 1973), so all clinical tests are needed to declare brain death and are likely essential.

Spinal reflexes may sometimes be present but they are not relevant in establishing brain death. Isolated clinical studies, electroencephalographic (EEG) examination and even blood flow determination, fall short of an absolute diagnosis of cerebral death.

Repetitive studies of a single functional system provide greater confidence but the time period is long and many patients die of cardiac arrest before they meet the criteria for cerebral death (George 1991). Within limits, the shorter the period of observation the more individuals may be diagnosed as cerebrally dead (Smith 1973), so after the first rapid evaluation, the clinical data should be confirmed by the following tests:
- conventional or CT angiography which shows no intracerebral filling at the level of the carotid bifurcation or Circle of Willis, patency of the external carotid circulation, and a delay in the filling of the superior longitudinal sinus (Brodac 1974; Frampas 2009),
- electroencephalography which shows no electrical activity for at least 30 minutes of recording in suspected brain death, as adopted by the American Electroencephalographic Society (Benett 1978), including 16 channel electroencephalographic instruments,
- transcranial Doppler ultrasonography; ten per cent of patients may not have temporal insonation windows, therefore the initial absence of Doppler signals cannot be interpreted as consistent with brain death; small systolic peaks in early systole without diastolic flow or reverberating flow, indicating very high vascular resistance associated with greatly increased intracranial pressure (Ropper 1987),
- technetium 99m hexamethyl propylene amineoxime brain scan: no uptake of isotope in brain (Hollow skull phenomenon),
- somatosensory evoked potentials which showed bilateral absence of N20-P23 response with median nerve stimulation, and its recordings should adhere to the minimal technical

criteria for somatosensory evoked potentials recording in suspected brain death as adopted by the American electrophysiological society (Benett 1978).

Conclusion

A neurological intensive care unit requires a multidisciplinary approach to the management of critically ill patients. The intensivists' and neurologists' attention to communication, daily nursing care, physical therapy, and infection control will ensure the best outcome (Rivers 2001).

9. Medical Diseases and Metabolic Encephalopathies
SAher HAshem, NAbil Kitchener

Neurological emergencies in medical diseases (secondary brain injury), e.g., renal coma, hepatic coma, salt and water imbalance, disturbance of glucose metabolism, other endocrinal causes of coma, disturbances of calcium and magnesium metabolism, drugs and intoxication, represent a good part of the patient population in the neurocritical care unit. Understanding the underlying mechanisms of secondary brain injury which include hypoxia, hypoperfusion, reperfusion injury with free radical formations, release of excitatory amino acids and harmful mediators from injured cells, and electrolyte and acid base changes from systemic or regional ischemia, are very important for proper management of such conditions. Management rules will be specified according to each cause and pathogenesis.

Metabolic encephalopathies are a group of neurological deficits affecting the brain causing delirium, confusion, or coma, caused by different mechanisms involving toxin production or interference with metabolic biochemical processes. Metabolic encephalopathies are usually multifactorial in origin, and are important complications of many diseases of patients treated in critical care units. Confusion is clinically defined as the inability to maintain a coherent stream of thought or action. Delirium is a confusional state with superimposed hyperactivity of the sympathetic limb of the autonomic nervous system with consequent signs including tremor, tachycardia, diaphoresis, and mydriasis. Acute toxic-metabolic encephalopathy (TME), which encompasses delirium and the acute confusional state, is an acute condition of global cerebral dysfunction in the absence of primary structural brain disease (Chen 1996).

Examination of the Encephalopathic Patient

1. Mental state assessment
    a. Level of consciousness using Glasgow Coma Scale (GCS),
    b. Memory and attention by Mini-Mental State Examination (MMSE),
    c. Mood (depression, elation, mania or irritability),
    d. Hallucination, which is usually visual.
2. Physical examination
    a. Temperature,
    b. Pulse (for tachycardia),
    c. Pupillary dysfunctions and extraocular movements, N.B. pupillary functions are ones that last and resist changes in metabolic encephalopathies.
    d. Respiratory pattern,
    e. Motor response,
    N.B. during examination of motor response look for presence of asterixis, which are drops of fully extended wrists for less than one second with re-extension again.
3. Investigations
    a. CSF examination,
    b. Full metabolic scanning of the blood,
    c. Neurophysiologic tests, e.g., EEG, evoked potentials,
        i. EEG patterns in metabolic encephalopathies are not specific (e.g., triphasic waves in hepatic encephalopathy). On the other hand, multifocal spikes are specific to lithium intoxication (Kaplan 2011).
        ii. Brain stem auditory evoked potentials (BAER) are resistant to metabolic changes.
    d. Neuroimaging, e.g., CT scan, MRI.

General Pathophysiology

Normal neuronal activity requires a balanced environment of electrolytes, water, amino acids, excitatory and inhibitory neurotransmitters, and metabolic substrates (Earnest 1993). In addition, normal blood flow, normal temperature, normal osmolality, and physiologic pH are required for optimal central nervous system function. Complex systems, including those mediating arousal and awareness and those involved in higher cognitive functions, are more likely to malfunction when the local body environment is deranged (Young 1998).

All forms of acute metabolic encephalopathy (ME) interfere with the function of the ascending reticular activating system and its projections to the cerebral cortex, leading to impairment of arousal and awareness. Ultimately, the neurophysiologic mechanisms of ME include interruption of polysynaptic pathways and altered excitatory-inhibitory amino acid balance (Lipton 1994). The pathophysiology of ME varies according to the underlying etiology.

Hepatic Encephalopathy

Hepatic encephalopathy (HE) appears as a complication of fulminant hepatic failure (FHF) and in chronic liver failure. Initially it is characterized by minor mental and personality changes with some cognitive impairment. With disease progression there are obvious motor abnormalities and increasing loss of consciousness until deep coma.

Etiology of fulminant hepatic failure includes viruses, drugs (such as halothane, acetaminophen, valproate and INH), and

acute fatty liver in pregnancy, toxins (such as amatoxins and phosphorus), Wilson disease and Rye's syndrome.

Pathophysiology of hepatic encephalopathy includes

neurotoxins (like ammonia, short- and medium-chain fatty acids, mercaptans, phenols, etc), and altered neurotransmission (due to benzodiazepine-like substances, and neurotransmitters' hypothesis including 5-HT and glutaminergic transmission). This may end in cerebral edema (Young 1998).

All of the following conditions may precipitate hepatic encephalopathy:
- Increased GIT protein absorption like in GIT hemorrhage or increased dietary protein
- Drugs like benzodiazepines or INH
- Renal dysfunction
- Catabolic states like infections and surgery
- Dehydration, hypokalemia, constipation
- Chronic hepatopathies which can present with FHF, e.g., cirrhosis with portal hypertension, portal vein thrombosis, Wilson disease, ornithine carbamoyltransferase deficiency and chronic valproate hepatopathy

Complications of hepatic encephalopathy (HE)

Epilepsy may complicate hepatic encephalopathy in 10–30% of cases, related to hypoglycemia. Cerebral edema may complicate hepatic encephalopathy in 80% of cases. Bleeding and renal dysfunction (i.e., renal failure in presence of normal-sized kidney (hepatorenal syndrome), with urine sodium concentration below 20 mmol/L, while the urine is hyperosmolar) may complicate hepatic encephalopathy also.

This syndrome is reversible with normalization of renal functions. Another form of renal dysfunction is pre-renal azotemia. Hypotension and derangement of acid base balance with acidosis is reported with cerebral edema and alkalosis, and is found with vomiting and hypokalaemia in cases of hepatic encephalopathy.

Table 9.1 – Differences between FHF and chronic hepatic encephalopathy

Feature	FHF	Chronic HE
History		
Onset	Acute	Insidious or subacute
Mental state	Mania → coma	Blunted → coma
Precipitation	Viral infection or hepatoxin	GIT hemorrhage, exogenous protein, uremia
History of liver disease	No	Yes
Symptoms		
Nausea & vomiting	Common	Unusual
Signs		
Liver	Small, soft, tender	Large, firm, painless
Nutritional state	Normal	Cachectic
Ascitis	Absent	May be present
Lab tests		
Transaminases	Very high	Normal or slightly high
Coagulopathy	Present	Often present

Table 9.2 – Clinical staging of hepatic encephalopathy

Grade	Consciousness	Intellect	Behavior	Motor	Psychometric
0-1	Normal	Normal	Normal	Normal	Poor performance
1	Inverted sleep Insomnia Hypersomnia	Short attention Low perception Impaired calculation	Anxiety Apathy Irritability Low monotonous voice	Incoordination Poor hand writing Tremors	Prolonged
2	Slow response Lethargy	Disorientation for time	Disinhibition Disobedience	Asterixis Ataxia Dysarthria Hyperreflexia	Very prolonged
3	Confusion Delirium Paranoia Semistupor	Disorientation for place Amnesia Perseverate	Bizarre behavior	Hyperreflexia Nystagmus Rigidity Yawing Incontinence	Unable to perform
4	Coma, arousal to pain Coma unresponsive	None	absent	Decorticate / Decerebrate posturing	Unable to perform

Treatment of hepatic encephalopathy

Fulminant Hepatic Failure (FHF). First of all, patients must be nourished by intravenous infusion of glucose 20–40%, then be given retention enema with 250 ml lactulose in 750 ml electrolyte solution, neomycin 2 g 2-3x daily, along with fresh frozen plasma (FFP) for coagulopathy. Plasma exchange can be used daily, until the prothrombin time is near normal (Quick score prolonged below 25%) or patient is awake. Hypotension must be treated with volume expanders. GIT bleeding is the second cause of death in FHF, administration of H_2 antagonists or proton pump inhibitors may help. Cerebral edema is treated by 20% manitol, 100 ml every 8 hours in absence of renal failure, but steroids are contraindicated. In cases of metabolic encephalopathy due to organ failure, transplantation may be an option. In In case of acetaminophen-induced fulminant hepatic failure, gastric lavage, forced diarrhea and N-acetyl cysteine infusion of 150 mg/kg diluted with glucose solution may help.

Hepatic encephalopathy in chronic liver disease. Most porto-systemic encephalopathies (PSE) occur as a consequence of dietary mistakes, GIT bleeding, hemorrhage, infection, alkalosis or hypokalemia as a result of diuretic therapy.

Hepatic encephalopathy in this case can be managed by a diet restricted in proteins, allow 30-40 g/day. Lactulose can be given at about 60-180 ml, in divided doses, to give 2-3 soft stools daily. In addition, neomycin (2 g twice daily) and flumazenil (a benzodiazepine receptor antagonist) should be given in 2 mg dose infused in 15 minutes (Onyekwere 2011).

Renal Encephalopathies

The most disabling feature of both renal failure and dialysis is encephalopathy. It is probably caused by the accumulation of renal toxins. Other important causes are related to the underlying disorders that cause renal failure, particularly hypertension. The clinical manifestations of renal (uremic) encephalopathy spans from mild confusional states to deep

coma, and movement disorders such as asterixis may be associated. Cognitive impairment is considered to be the major indication for the initiation of renal dialysis with or without subsequent transplantation. Sleep disorders including restless legs syndrome are also common in patients with kidney failure. Renal dialysis is also associated with neurologic complications including acute dialysis encephalopathy and chronic dialysis encephalopathy, formerly known as dialysis dementia (Seifter 2011).

Five major syndromes of CNS affection are seen in renal failure.
- Acute renal failure: asterixis, myoclonus, seizures, irritability and raised deep tendon reflexes.
- Chronic renal failure: early personality changes, polyneuropathy.
- Dialysis disequilibrium syndrome: usually when there is rapid hemodialysis, it presents by headache, lethargy, nausea and vomiting.
- Chronic dialysis encephalopathy (dialysis dementia): always late in the course of chronic renal failure. It gives dysarthria, deterioration in memory, progressing to myoclonus, mutism, coma and death (Seifter 2011).
- Renal transplantation: patients with renal transplantation may experience encephalopathy (soon) after transplantation. Immunosuppressive drugs, like cyclosporine and acyclovir may produce confusion, lethargy and coma at toxic levels. (Later) after transplantation, primary CNS lymphoma becomes a major concern in patients developing symptoms of brain dysfunction.

Management of acute and chronic renal failure is by hemodialysis; dialysis disequilibrium syndrome is managed by prolonging the time of dialysis; management of chronic dialysis encephalopathy is by renal transplantation.

Fluid and Electrolyte Imbalance

Osmolarity disorders

Hypernatremia: Hypernatremia indicates a deficit of body water relative to sodium concentration. Clinically, it is similar to hyponatremia where encephalopathy possibly develops, due to dehydration. Usually, hypernatremic patients are hypovolemic. Common causes of hyponatremia are

- Pure water loss (in renal diabetes insipidus and external insensible losses via the skin and lungs).
- Combined water and sodium loss (in renal osmotic diuresis combined with inadequate water intake, and external excessive sweating).
- Inadequate sodium gain (in cases of excessive sodium administration, like hypertonic solutions; adrenal hyperfunction, like hyperaldosteronism, Cushing Syndrome; and intake of exogenous steroids).

Hypernatremia should be corrected slowly. When volume depletion with circulatory insufficiency is predominant, vigorous treatment with isotonic saline solution is mandatory. When the cause is diabetes insipidus, administer 2-5 units of aqueous vasopressin, or 1-5 mcg of desmopressin (DDAVP) should be given subcutaneously or intranasally. When hypernatremia is due to excessive gain, hypotonic (0.45%) saline is used to replace, in part, additional water deficits.

Hyponatremia: Three types of hyponatremia are described:

Hypovolemic hyponAtremiA: patients with low intake of sodium-containing fluids and have attempted replacement with free water may present with encephalopathy.

Hypervolemic hyponAtremiA: usually seen in congestive heart failure or hypoalbuminemia. This condition can be treated with fluid restriction, a wise use of diuretics as well as treatment of the primary cause.

Euvolemic hyponatremia: This condition is seen in syndromes of inappropriate secretion of ADH (SIADH) adrenal insufficiency, hypothyroidism, severe psychogenic polydipsia, and hypoglycemia; also in pancreatitis with hyperlipidemia and hyperproteinemia. The degree of encephalopathy produced by hyponatremia depends on the rate of fall of serum sodium rather than its value.

All cases of euvolemic hyponatremia are treated with fluid restriction (800-1000 ml/d) and removal of precipitants (Young 1998).

Central pontine myelinolysis (CPM): Due to rapid correction of hyponatremia by more than 10 meq/d. Clinically, patients present with quadriparesis and cranial nerve dysfunction over several days, which may be followed by encephalopathy. The maximal lesion is seen in the basis pontis, but supratentorial white matter is also affected.

Syndrome of inappropriate secretion of antidiuretic hormone (SIADH): It is a common syndrome in neurological diseases; it leads to hyponatremia and increases salt concentration in urine (>20 mmol/L). Serum ADH is high. Causes of SIADH include

- Malignant neoplasms likes oat-cell carcinoma of lung, and Hodgkin disease
- Non-malignant pulmonary diseases, e.g., TB, emphysema, pneumothorax
- CNS diseases like subarachnoid hemorrhage, cerebral venous thrombosis, encephalitis, and meningitis, and PNS diseases like Guillain-Barré syndrome.
- Use of drugs like vincristine, carbamazepine, tricyclic antidepressants, etc.

Slow correction of hyponatremia by IV 3% sodium solution is recommended. IV 100 cc given over one-hour interval, until serum sodium level reach 125 mmol/l. Do not exceed correction rate of 2 mmol/h.

Hypercalcemia: The encephalopathy of hypercalcemia is not different from any metabolic encephalopathy except in early anosmia.

Other findings in hypercalcemia are myopathy, polyuria, pruritis, nausea and vomiting. Patients start to complain at serum calcium level of 13 mg/dl, when abnormal EEG changes start to appear. Patients suffering from hyperparathyroidism may manifest seizures independent of serum calcium level due to elevated serum parathormone.

Management: Hypercalcemia is corrected by saline diuresis, augmented with furosemide, followed by a choice of mithramycin steroids, phosphate or etidronate.

Encephalopathy in Diabetic Patients

Hypoglycemia: Clinically, patients who develop hypoglycemia are graded:
- At 20 mg/dl, immediate loss of consciousness in adults and children, neonates resist hypoglycemia better,
- At 45 mg/dl, confusion, irritability. Sometimes unexplained focal lesions appear with hypoglycemia.

Management: give IV glucose at 1 g/kg body weight, plus thiamine 1 mg/kg to prevent Wernicke's encephalopathy (Quinn 2002).

Nonketotic hyperosmolar hyperglycemia (NHH): Usually occurs in diabetic patients whose insulin production is adequate to inhibit lipolysis, but insufficient to prevent hyperglycemia, which result in a marked osmotic diuresis. Diuresis leads to dehydration and hyperosmolarity. In such situations, serum glucose may rise to 800-1200 mg/dl, and serum osmolarity may exceed 350 mOsm/L, which may invite development of brain edema.

Osmolarity= $2(Na+K) + (glucose/18) + (BUN/2.8)$

Clinically, patients present with encephalopathy, focal

neurological signs, and partial seizures that do not respond to conventional antiepileptic medication. Such encephalopathy must be treated by rehydration.

Management: Normal saline is infused slowly to correct hypotension and improve osmolality, in addition to insulin

infusion at the rate of 10 IU/h, with regular checking of plasma glucose, since these patients are very sensitive to insulin.

Glucose should be added to saline when plasma glucose is approximately 300 mg/dl (Quinn 2002).

Diabetic ketoacidosis (DKA): About 80% of DKA patients have encephalopathy and 10% are comatose. Management: Like NHH, but with higher amounts of insulin. If there is evidence of brain edema mannitol is used. If there is evidence of electrolyte imbalance, mandate correction. The use of IV sodium bicarbonate to compensate for metabolic acidosis is debatable (Quinn 2002).

Hypoxic Ischemic Encephalopathy (HIE)

Following cardiac or respiratory arrest, CO poisoning or cyanide poisoning, one of four clinical syndromes might appear:
- Global encephalopathy
- Memory loss
- Postanoxic Parkinsonism
- Lance-Adams syndrome (intention myoclonus)

Findings predicting good prognosis are preserved pupillary responses, preserved roving eye movement, decorticate posture or better at initial examination. We predict good prognosis when we find in clinical examination after 24 hours, motor withdrawal from noxious stimuli or improvement of 2 grades in eye movement. Also, finding motor withdrawal or better, and normal spontaneous eye movements at 72 hours examination, carries a good prognosis. Also, when a patient obeys commands at the 1-

week examination.

Management is by hyperventilation and osmotic diuresis, for cerebral edema. Seizure control is live saving and has an impact on prognosis, as patients suffering from GTCS have a better outcome than those who suffer from myoclonic seizures.

Septic Encephalopathy

Septic encephalopathy is a frequent sequel of severe sepsis, with no definite therapeutic strategies available that can prevent associated neurological dysfunction and damage. It is caused by a number of processes, such as direct bacterial invasion, toxic effects of endotoxins, inflammatory mediators, impairment of microcirculation, and neuroendocrine changes. The exact cellular and molecular mechanisms remain an enigma. Several mediators of inflammation have been assigned a key role in etiogenesis of encephalopathy, including cytokines, chemokines and complement cascade. With the observations that brain dysfunction in such sepsis disorders can be alleviated by regulation of the cytokines and complements in various species of animals, optimism is building for a possible therapy of the sepsis-damaged brain (Jacob 2011).

Early aggressive treatment with antibiotics is key, along with modulators of cytokines and complements and anti-inflammatory medicines (Jacob 2011).

Drug-induced Encephalopathies

Commonly implicated drugs in encephalopathy etiology include salicylates, tricyclic antidepressants, lithium, sedatives, neuroleptics, methyldopa, amantadine, acyclovir, digitalis, propranolol, hydantoins, etc (Jain 2001).

Drug-induced delirium results from disruption of the normal integration of neurotransmitters, including dopamine, acetylcholine, glutamate, gamma-aminobutyric acid (GABA), and/or serotonin (Young 1998).

10. References

Adams HP, del Zoppo G, Alberts MJ, et al. Guidelines for the Early Management of Adults With Ischemic Stroke. Circulation 2007;115:e478-534.

Adams RE, Powers WJ. Management of hypertension in acute critical ill patients. Crit Care Clin 1997;13:131-61.

Amin DK, Shah PK, Swan HJ. Deciding when hemodynamic monitoring is appropriate. J Crit Illn 1993;8:1053-61.

Anaesthesia UK, 2011. (Accessed July 19, 2011, at http://www.frca.co.uk). Andrew B. Intracranial Pressure and Cerebral Blood Flow Monitoring. In:
Neurocritical care. Michael Torbey ed. 2010:109-118. Cambridge Books Online, Cambridge University Press (Accessed June 24, 2011, at http://dx.doi.org/10.1017/CBO9780511635434).

Arnow P, Quimosing E, Beach M. Consequences of intravascular sepsis. Clin infect Dis 1993;16:778–84.

Badley EM. An introduction to the concepts and classification of impairments, disabilities and handicaps. Disabil Rehabil 1993;19:161-78.

Baldwin K, Orr S, Briand M, Piazza C, Veydt A, McCoy S. Acute ischemic stroke update. Pharmacotherapy 2010;30:493-514.

Bamford J. Clinical examination in diagnosis and subclassification of stroke. Lancet 1992;339:400-2.

Bassin S, Smith TL, Bleck TP. Clinical review: status epilepticus. Crit Care 2002;6:137-42.

Bateman DE. Neurological assessment of coma. J Neurol Neurosurgery Psychiatry 2001;71:i13-7.

Benett DR. The EEG in determination of brain death. Ann NY Acad Sci 1978;315:110-20.

Berg K, Maki B, Williams JI, Holliday P, Wood-Dauphinee S. Clinical and laboratory measures of postural balance in an elderly population. Arch Phys Med Rehabil 1992;73:1073-83.

Bergner M, Bobbitt RA, Carter WB, et al. The Sickness Impact Profile: development and final revision of a health status measure. Med Care 1981;19:787-805.

Bernard GR, Artigas A, Brigham KL, et al. The American-European consensus conference on ARDS, definitions, mechanisms, relevant outcomes, and clinical trials co-ordination. Am J Respir Crit Care Med 1994;149:818–24.

Blanchard AR. Sedation and analgesia in intensive care. Medications attenuate stress response in critical illness. Postgrad Med 2002;111:59–70.

Bonita R, Beaglehole R. Recovery of motor function after stroke. Stroke 1988;19:1497-500.

Borel CO. Neurologic intensive care unit catastrophes: airway, breathing, and circulation. Current Treatment Options in Neurology 2000;2:499-506.

Brain Trauma Foundation Guidelines 2007. (Accessed July 21, 2011, at http://www.braintrauma.org).

Brodac G B, Smmon RS. Angiography in brain death neuroradiology 1974;7:25-8.

Brott T, Adams HP, Olinger CP, et al. Measurements of acute cerebral infarction: a clinical examination scale. Stroke 1989;20:864-70.

Campbell AJ, Cook JA, Adey G, Cuthbertson BH. Predicting death and readmission after intensive care discharge. Br J Anaesth 2008;100:656-62.

Cecil S, Chen PM, Callaway SE, Rowland SM, Adler DE, Chen JW. Traumatic brain injury: advanced multimodal neuromonitoring from theory to clinical practice. Crit Care Nurse 2011;31:25-36.

Chen R, Young GB. Metabolic Encephalopathies. In: Bolton, CF, Young, GB, eds. Baillere's Clinical Neurology. Balliere Tindall, London 1996:

577-92. Clark WC, Muhlbauer MS, Lowery R, Hartman M, Ray MW, Watridge CB.

Complications of intracranial pressure monitoring in trauma patients. Neurosurgery 1989;25:20-4.

Collen FM, Wade DT, Robb GF, Bradshaw CM. The Rivermead Mobility Index: a further development of the Rivermead Motor Assessment. Int Disabil Stud 1991;13:50-4.

Collen FM, Wade DT, Bradshaw CM. Mobility after stroke: reliability of measures of impairment and disability. Int Disabil Stud 1990;12:6-9.

Collin C, Wade D. Assessing motor impairment after stroke: a pilot reliability study. J Neurol Neurosurg Psychiatry 1990;53:576-9.

Cote R, Hachinski VC, Shurvell BL, Norris JW, Wolfson C. The Canadian Neurological Scale: a preliminary study in acute stroke. Stroke 1986;17:731-7.

Crutchfeld JS, Narayan RK, Robertson CS, Michael LH. Evaluation of a fiberoptic intracranial pressure monitor. J Neurosurg 1990;72:482-7.

Cunningham C, Horgan F, and O'Neill. Clinical assessment of rehabilitation potential of older patients: a pilot study. Clin Rehabil 2000:14:205-7.

Curley FJ, Smyrnios NS. Routine Monitoring of Critically Ill Patients. J Intensive Care Med 1990;4:153-74.

Czosnyka M, Guazzo E, Whitehouse M, et al. Significance of intracranial pressure waveform analysis after head injury. Acta Neurochir 1996;138:531-42.

Czosnyka M, Kirkpatrick PJ, Pickard JD. Multimodal monitoring and assessment of cerebral hemodynamic reserve after severe head injury. Cerbrovasc Brain Metab Rev 1996;8:273-95.

Czosnyka M, Pickard JD. Monitoring and interpretation of intracranial pressure. J Neurol Neurosurg Psychiatry 2004;75:813-21.

Czosnyka M, Richards HK, Czosnyka Z, Piechnik S, Pickard JD. Vascular components of cerebrospinal fluid compensation. J Neurosurg 1999;90:752-9.

Daly K, Beale R, Chang RWS. Reduction in mortality after inappropriate early discharge from intensive care unit: logistic regression triage model. BMJ 2001;322:1274-6.

Domingues RB, Tsanaclis AM, Pannuti CS, Mayo MS, Lakeman FD. Evaluation of the range of clinical presentations of herpes simplex encephalitis by using polymerase chain reaction assay of cerebrospinal fluid samples. Clin Infect Dis 1997;25:86-91.

Earnest MP, Parker WD. Metabolic encephalopathies and coma from medical causes. In: Grotta J, eds. Management of the Acutely Ill Neurological Patient. Churchill Livingstone, New York 1993:1-18.

Egol A, Fromm R, Guntupalli KK, et al. Guidelines for intensive care unit admission, discharge, and triage. Crit Care Med 1999;27:633-8.

Fagon JY, Chastre J, Hance A, et al. Nosocomial pneumonia in ventilated patients: a cohort study evaluating attributable mortality and hospital stay. Am J Med 1993;94:281-8.

Fjærtoft H, Rohweder G, Indredavik B. Stroke unit care combined with early supported discharge improves 5-year outcome: a randomized controlled trial. Stroke 2011;42:1707-11.

Folstein MF, Folstein SE, McHugh PR. "Mini-mental state". A practical method for grading the cognitive state of patients for the clinician. J Psychiatr Res 1975;12:189-98.

Formisano R, Carlesimo GA, Sabbadini M. Clinical predictors and neuropsychological outcome in severe traumatic brain injury patients. Acta Neurochir 2004;146:457–62.

Frampas E, Videcoq M, de Kerviler E, et al. CT angiography for brain death diagnosis. AJNR Am J Neuroradiol 2009;30:1566-70.

Fugl-Meyer AR, Jaasko L, Leyman I, Olsson S, Steglind S. The post stroke hemiplegic patient. A method for evaluation of physical performance. Scand J Rehabil Med 1975;7:13-31.

García X, Pinsky MR. Clinical applicability of functional hemodynamic monitoring. Ann Intensive Care 2011;25:1-35.

George MS. Establishing brain death: the potential role of nuclear medicine in the search for reliable confirmatory test. Eu J Nucl Med 1991;18:75-7.

Goldberg S. The Four-Minute Neurologic Exam. Miami, MedMaster Inc., 1987. Gomes CAR, Lustosa SAS, Matos D, Andriolo RB, Waisberg DR, Waisberg J.
Percutaneous endoscopic gastrostomy versus nasogastric tube feeding for adults with swallowing disturbances. Cochrane Database Syst Rev 2010;11:CD008096.

Goodglass H, Kaplan E. Boston Diagnostic Aphasia Examination (BDAE). Philadelphia: Lea and Febiger, 1983.

Gopinath SP, Robertson CS, Contant CF et al. Jugular venous desaturation and outcome after head injury. J Neurol Neurosurg Psychiatry 1994;57:717-23.

Gupta AK. Monitoring the injured brain in the intensive care unit. J Postgrad Med 2002;48:218-25.

Hajjar K, Kerr DM, Lees KR. Thrombolysis for acute ischemic stroke. J Vasc Surg 2011;54:901-7.

Hand PJ, Kwan J, Lindley RI, Dennis MS, Wardlaw JM. Distinguishing between stroke and mimic at the bedside: the brain attack study. Stroke 2006;37:769-75.

Hardin KA, Seyal M, Stewart T, Bonekat HW. Sleep in critically ill chemically paralyzed patients requiring mechanical ventilation. Chest 2006;129:1468-77.

Hofmeijer J, Kappelle LJ, Algra A, et al. Surgical decompression for space-occupying cerebral infarction (the Hemicraniectomy After Middle Cerebral

Artery infarction with Life-threatening Edema Trial [HAMLET]): a multicentre, open, randomised trial. Lancet Neurol 2009;8:326-33.

Holmes JF, Palchak MJ, MacFarlane T, Kuppermann N. Performance of the pediatric Glasgow coma scale in children with blunt head trauma. Acad Emerg Med 2005;12:814-9.

Hurford WE. Sedation and paralysis during mechanical ventilation. Respir Care 2002;47:334-47.

Inouye SK, van Dyck CH, Alessi CA, Balkin S, Siegal AP, Horwitz RI. Clarifying confusion: the confusion assessment method. A new method for detection of delirium. Ann Intern Med 1990;113:941-8.

Inouye SK. Delirium in older persons. N Engl J Med 2006;354:1157-65.

Jacob A, Brorson JR, Alexander JJ. Septic encephalopathy: inflammation in man and mouse. Neurochem Int 2011;58:472-6.

Jacobi J, Fraser GL, Coursin DB, et al. Clinical practice guidelines for the sustained use of sedatives and analgesics in the critically ill adult. Crit care Med 2002;30:119-41.

Jain KK, Bradley WG. Drug-Induced Neurological Disorders. Second Edition. Hogrefe & Huber Publishers, 2001.

Joseph M. Intracranial pressure monitoring: vital information ignored. Indian J Crit Care Med 2005;9:35-41.

Juul N, Morris GF, Marshall SB, Marshall LF. Intracranial hypertension and cerebral perfusion pressure: influence on neurological deterioration and outcome in severe head injury. The executive committee of international selfotel trial. J Neurosurg 2000;92:1-6.

Kaplan PW, Rossetti AO. EEG patterns and imaging correlations in encephalopathy: encephalopathy part II. J Clin Neurophysiol 2011;28:233-51.

Kertesz A. Western Aphasia Battery. New York: Grune & Stratton, 1982.

Kiernan RJ, Mueller J, Langston JW, Van Dyke C. The Neurobehavioral Cognitive
Status Examination: a brief but quantitative approach to cognitive assessment. Ann Intern Med 1987;107:481-5.

Kitchener N, Zakieldine H, Abdelkarim A, Ghoraba MA, Helmy S. Non-convulsive status epilepticus in ischemic stroke and its impact on prognosis. J Neurol 2010;257:S1-S246 (abstract).

Leon Carrion J, VanEeckhout P, Dominguez, Morales M. The locked in syndrome. Brain injury 2002;16:555-69.

Levin MJ, Weinberg A, Sandberg E, Sylman J, Tyler KL. Atypical herpes simplex virus encephalitis diagnosed by PCR amplification of viral DNA from CSF. Neurology 1998;51:554-9.

Lewis L, Miller D, Morley J, et al. Unrecognized delirium in ED geriatric patients.

Am J Emerg Med 1995;13:142-145.

Lipton SA, Rosenberg PA. Excitatory amino acids as a final common pathway for neurologic disorders. N Engl J Med 1994;330:613.

Mahoney FI, Barthel DW. Functional evaluation: the Barthel Index. Maryland State Med J 1965;14:61-5.

Manno EM. New management strategies in the treatment of status epilepticus Mayo Clinic Proc 2003;78:508-18.

Marmarou A, Anderson RL, Ward JD, et al. Impact of ICP instability and hypotension on outcome in patients with severe head trauma. J Neurosurg 1991;75:S59-S66.

Mathew NT, Meyer JS, Rivera VM, Charney JZ, Hartmann A. Double-blind evaluation of glycerol therapy in acute cerebral infarction. Lancet 1972;2:1327-1329.

McMillian WD, Taylor S, Lat I. Sedation, analgesia, and delirium in the critically ill patient. J Pharm Pract 2011;24:27-34.

Mistri AK, Robinson TG, Potter JF. Pressor therapy in acute ischemic stroke: systematic review. Stroke 2006;36:1565-71.

Monkhouse S. CRANIAL NERVES: Functional Anatomy. Cambridge University Press, New York, USA, 2006.

Moppett IK, Mahajan RP. Transcranial Doppler ultrasonography in anaesthesia and intensive care. Br J Anaesth 2004;93:710-724.

Murray MJ, Cowen J, Deblock H, etal. Clinical practice guidelines for sustained neuromuscular blockade in the adult critically ill patients. Crit Care Med 2002;30:142-56.

Oddo M, Levine JM, Frangos S, et al. Effect of mannitol and hypertonic saline on cerebral Oxygenation in patients with severe traumatic brain injury and refractory intracranial hypertension. J Neurol Neurosurg Psychiatry 2009;80:916–20.

Onyekwere CA, Ogbera AO, Hameed L. Chronic liver disease and hepatic encephalopathy: Clinical profile and outcomes. Niger J Clin Pract 2011;14:181-5.

Owen-Reece H, Smith M, Elwell CE, Goldstone JC. Near Infrared spectroscopy. Br J Anaesth 1999;82:418-26.

Pelosi P, Ferguson ND, Frutos-Vivar F, et al. Management and outcome of mechanically ventilated neurologic patients. Crit Care Med 2011;39:1482- 92.

Pincus SM. Approximate entropy as a measure of system complexity. Proc Natl Acad Sci USA 1991;15:88;2297-301.

Plum F, Posner JB, Saper CB, Schiff ND. Plum and Posner's diagnosis of stupor and coma. Fourth Edition. Published by Oxford University Press Inc, 2007.

Poole JL, Whitney SL. Motor assessment scale for stroke patients: concurrent validity and interrater reliability. Arch Phys Med Rehabil 1988;69:195-7.

Porch B. Porch Index of Communicative Ability (PICA). Palo Alto: Consulting Psychologists Press; 1981.

Quinn L. Pharmacologic treatment of the critically ill patient with diabetes. Crit Care Nurs Clin North Am 2002;14:81-98.

Rankin J. Cerebral vascular accidents in patients over the age of 60. Scott Med J 1957;2:200-15.

Raslan A, Bhardwaj A. Medical management of cerebral edema. Neurosurg Focus 2007;22:E12.

Rivers E, Nguyen B, Havstad S, et al. Early goal-directed therapy in the treatment of severe sepsis and septic shock. N Engl J Med 2001;345:1368–77.

Ropper A H, Kehene S M, Wechsler L. Transcranial Doppler in brain death. Neurology 1987;37:1733-35.

Sakr Y, Vincent JL, Reinhart K, et al. Use of the pulmonary artery catheter is not associated with worse outcome in the ICU. Chest 2005;128:2722-31.

Schnakers C, Zasler ND. Pain assessment and management in disorders of consciousness. Curr Opin Neurol 2007;20:620-6.

Seifter JL, Samuels MA. Uremic encephalopathy and other brain disorders associated with renal failure. Semin Neurol 2011;31:139-43.

Semplicini A, Maresca A, Boscolo G. Hypertension in acute ischemic stroke: a compensatory mechanism or an additional damaging factor. Arch Intern Med 2003;163:211-6.

Sessler CN, Gosnell MS, Grap MJ, et al. The Richmond Agitation–Sedation Scale: Validity and Reliability in Adult Intensive Care Unit Patients. Am J Respir Crit Care Med 2002;166:1338-44.

Shoemaker WC, Parsa MH. Invasive and noninvasive monitoring. In: Textbook of critical care. Fourth Edition. Ayres SM, Grenvik A, Holbrook P, Shoemaker
W.C. Eds. Philadelphia, WB Saunders 2000;74-7.

Shorvon SD. Status epilepticus: its clinical features and treatment in children and adults. Cambridge: Cambridge University Press, 1994.

Smith AJ, Walker AF. Cerebral blood flow and brain metabolism as indicators of cerebral death: a review. Johns Hopkins Med J 1973;133:107-19.

Stasiukyniene V, Pilvinis V, Reingardiene D, Janauskaite L. Epileptic seizures in critically ill patients. Medicina 2009;45:501-7.

Steiger HJ, Aaslid R, Stooss R, Seiler RW. Transcranial Doppler monitoring in head injury: relations between type of injury, flow velocities, vasoreactivity, and outcome. Neurosurgery 1994;34:79-85.

Stevens RD, Bhardwaj A. Approach to the comatose patient. Crit Care Med 2006;34:31-41.

Strub RL, Black FW. The Mental Status Examination, 4th Edition. FA Davis Co., Philadelphia, 2000.

Teasdale G, Jennett B. Assessment of coma and impaired consciousness: a practical scale. Lancet 1974;2:81-4.

Teasdale G, Murray G, Parker L, Jennett B. Adding up the Glasgow Coma Scale. Acta Neurochir 1979;28:13-6.

Thuriaux MC. The ICIDH: evolution, status, and prospects. Disabil Rehabil 1995;17:112-8.

Upchurch GR, Demling RH, Davies J, Gates JD, Knox JB. Efficacy of subcutaneous heparin in prevention of venous thromboembolic events in trauma patients. Am Surg 1995;61:749-55.

Valles J, Leon C, Alvarez-Lerma F. Nosocomial bacteraemia in critically ill patients: a multicentre study evaluating epidemiology and prognosis. Clin Infect Dis 1997;24:387–95.

Van Swieten JC, Koudstaal PJ, Visser MC, Schouten HJ, van Gijn J. Interobserver agreement for the assessment of handicap in stroke patients. Stroke 1988;19:604-7.

Vincent JL, Bihari DJ, Suter PM, et al. The prevalence of nosocomial infections in intensive care units in Europe: results of the EDPIC study. JAMA 1995;274:639–44.

Wade DT, Collin C. The Barthel ADL Index: a standard measure of physical disability? Int Disabil Stud 1988;10:64-7.

Wade DT, de jong BA. Recent advances in rehabilitation. BMJ 2000;320:1385-8. Walley KR. Use of Central Venous Oxygen Saturation to Guide Therapy. Am J

Respir Crit Care Med 2011;184:514-20.

Wanklyn P, Cox N, Belfield P. Outcome in patients who require a gastrostomy after stroke. Age Ageing 1995;24:510-4.

Ware JE, Sherbourne CD. The MOS 36-Item short-form health survey (SF-36). I. Conceptual framework and item selection. Med Care 1992;30:473-83.

Webb AR, Singer M. Respiratory monitoring. In: Webb AR, Shapiro MJ, Singer M, et al, eds. Oxford textbook of critical care. Oxford: Oxford University Press, 1999:120-126.

Wijdicks EF. Brain death worldwide: accepted fact but no global consensus in diagnostic criteria. Neurology 2002;58:20-5.

Wijdicks E, Bamlet WR, Maramatton BV, Manno EM, McClelland RL. Validation of a new coma scale: The FOUR Score. Ann Neurol 2005;58:585-93.

Wood KE, Becker BN, McCartney JG: Care of the potential organ donor. N Eng JMed 2004;351:2730-9.

World Stroke Organization (WSO). World Stroke Organization declares public health emergency on World Stroke Day 2010. Accessed on August 15, 2011 at (http://goo.gl/alpn4).

Young GB, DeRubeis DA. Metabolic encephalopathies. In: Young GB, Ropper AH, Bolton CF, eds. Coma and Impaired Consciousness, McGraw-Hill 1998. p.307.

Young JS, Blow O, Turrentine F, Claridge JA, Schulman A. Is there an upper limit of intracranial pressure in patients with severe head injury if cerebral perfusion pressure is maintained? Neurosurg Focus 2003;15:E2.

Made in the USA
Coppell, TX
21 June 2022

79109365R00069